AUTISM – ONE FAMILY'S JOURNEY

First published 2022

Copyright © Velora M Levy Sailsman 2022

The right of Velora M Levy Sailsman to be identified as the author of this work has been asserted in accordance with the Copyright, Designs & Patents Act 1988.

All rights reserved. No part of this book may be reproduced, stored in a retrieval system, or transmitted in any form or by any means, electronic, electrostatic, magnetic tape, mechanical, photocopying, recording or otherwise, without the written permission of the copyright holder.

Published under licence by Brown Dog Books and
The Self-Publishing Partnership Ltd, 10b Greenway Farm, Bath Rd, Wick,
nr. Bath BS30 5RL

www.selfpublishingpartnership.co.uk

ISBN printed book: 978-1-83952-446-2
ISBN e-book: 978-1-83952-447-9

Cover design by Kevin Rylands
Internal design by Andrew Easton

Printed and bound in the UK

This book is printed on FSC certified paper

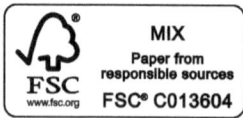

AUTISM – ONE FAMILY'S JOURNEY
A BOY CALLED ZEKE

VELORA M. LEVY-SAILSMAN

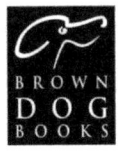

This book is dedicated to Zeke my ASD son, my husband Zephie, my first and second born Kelsey and Cuffie and to my two amazing granddaughters.

A special thank you to the family's GP, Dr Gloria Okafor, who took the care of Zeke's inner ear problems in hand.

Foreword 1: Natasha Gordon

Velora has a passion for helping children with autism thrive so they can reach their full potential. This has stemmed from her personal and professional experiences of managing children, including her own, with autism. I have seen her son progress tremendously in communication, hobbies and interests because of Velora's care and motivation. This book will support parents and carers by giving a greater depth of understanding, awareness of autism, the trials, struggles and successes that will inspire you to not give up.

Knowledge is power as they say! When parents first get the diagnosis that their child has autism, it can be very overwhelming and some parents carry the guilt, shame and emotional pain around with them due to lack of immediate support. In this book, Velora shares her experience, knowledge and expertise to improve your wellbeing and reduce your fears and anxieties. From reading this book I have gained further insight, knowledge and wisdom about autism. I have a greater admiration for Velora's strength and patience as well as her determination to be a good mother and wife despite her daily challenges.

Natasha Gordon: www.familywellness.org.uk

VELORA M. LEVY-SAILSMAN

Co-Author of 'Single mothers diary' | NCT Practitioner | Hypno-birthing Mindful Mamma Practitioner | Family Wellness Practitioner | Systematic Kinesiologist | Trauma Therapist

Forward 2: Ngozi Obanye

I first met Velora Levy-Sailsman and her son Zeke eight years ago at Haringey shed inclusive theatre company for young people of all abilities. They provide dance, drama and singing opportunities. Prior to my experience of meeting Velora, I had little understanding of autism. Since meeting Velora my knowledge and experience of the condition is now greatly increased. Coupled with her educational background and knowledge in special educational needs, she was able to develop and enhance coping strategies, as well as processing the myriad of emotions that she encountered on her autism journey. Velora experienced barriers to support services, communication issues with professionals and a general lack of awareness and understanding of autism within communities. These reasons enabled her to set up a C.I.C, Velora Autism Corner.

Velora Autism Corner (VAC) supports young people from the ages of 11 years to 25 years and their families and friends. They work with families and caregivers to understand the difficulties autistic young people face. They help them to overcome some of these challenges. They offer comprehensive support programmes of which include: Weekly youth club | Holiday scheme | Reading recovery | Home help | Youth minding/Respite | Independence training.

This book will help the layperson to gain an understanding into the world of autism instead of having a distorted view and also break down stigma. In some cultures, autism is seen as shame, annoyance, disappointment, regrets and antisocial. I remember a parent saying to me once, that her autistic daughter was labelled as 'disruptive'. Such negative attitudes can keep families from seeking the help they need and prevent them from enjoying the same quality of life as their neighbours. For families that have children with a diagnosis of autism, this book is positive, well informed and supportive. There are ideas in managing behavioural issues, including obsessive behaviour. Also working alongside mainstream schools and other establishments helps to develop individual needs, allowing Parents And caregivers to understand their particular talents and abilities.

Ngozi Obanye: www.edenjar.org.uk

Co-Author of '100 Years Unheard' – Poetry and Prose by the group, Afrikan Heritage Writers. Director of The Eden Jar-A Creativity-in Health Community Organisation.

Biography: THE BIO OF VELORA M. LEVY-SAILSMAN

Velora M. Levy-Sailsman was born in Jamaica. At age 14 years she moved to live in England. After finishing a turbulent secondary school experience in the West Midlands she moved to London in 1977 where she worked several jobs to maintain herself. She progressed onto receiving a college education between 1978 and 1983.

In 1983 she completed a 'Fresh Horizons' course at 'The City Lit' in Central London. Not only did this course elevate her education but it served as a therapy, equipping her with the confidence she needed to survive in a challenging world. In 1984 she commenced a Social Science Degree at Brunel University. After studying at Brunel for four years she graduated with Honours in Psychology.

In 1990 she progressed onto West London Institute of Higher Education (WLIH) where she completed the Post Graduate Certificate in Education (PGCE) and became a qualified Primary School teacher.

In 1997 she commenced studying for the qualification to become a teacher for children with a specific learning difficulty (SPLD), such as autism and dyslexia, which she successfully completed in 1999, after giving birth to her third child in 1998.

In 2001, her youngest child aged 3 years commenced having a series of tests to determine if he had autism and at age 6 years he was given the formal diagnosis. In order to become actively involved with the learning targets and strategies set for him by his school and other professionals, Velora established a small nursery for children as a means to supplement her husband's income. With the help of her dedicated staff, she successfully managed her nursery business for nine years.

In 2013 she decided to return to the classroom - this time, however, as a part-time Learning Support Teacher. With time on her hands during the days, while her youngest child was at school she decided to revisit the manuscript she had been working on haphazardly over a few years. In November 2016 she had her first book published, entitled *She caused the lightning to strike*. To date over 2000 copies of this book have been sold worldwide.

Autism - One family's journey - A boy called Zeke is Velora's second book. This book describes her journey of raising a child with autism.

In May 2018 she became the founder and Chief Executive Officer (CEO) of an organisation called 'Velora Autism Corner' which presently has six programmes assigned to it. The main ethos of this business is that it's for 'young people with autism' staffed by 'adults with autism'.

AUTISM – ONE FAMILY'S JOURNEY

ORGANISATIONS AND PEOPLE THAT HAVE HELPED ME COPE WITH THE PRESSURES FROM MY ASD CHILD:

Bowes Primary School
Hounsfield after school club
Raglan holiday play scheme
Tottenham Hotspurs Teen scheme
Team Spirit after school and holiday club
River Side athletics club and gym,
Albany swimming club for children with disabilities
Haringey Sixth Form College
Haringey Shed for dance/ singing
Leapfrog SPECIAL NEEDS play group
The light and sound THERAPY centre

Family members who have assisted with caring for Zeke after his diagnosis:

Zeke's father, my brother Oliver, my daughter Kelsey, my son Cuffie, and my son's fiancée Talia.

Zeke's support workers: Kieron , Elton, Immanuel, Albert and Nathaniel

Acknowledgements:
Readers of my manuscript:

Rebecca Turner (USA) Lawrence Goldstone (UK) Natasha Gordon (UK).

A special thank you to the above three wonderful people for investing their time to reading my manuscript.

CONTENTS

Introduction   19
Chapter 1 What is autism?   21
Recent data collected in several countries point to an increase in the number of children being diagnosed with autism

Chapter 2 The Autism spectrum
Dean Beadle discuss his views and experience of autism   27

Chapter 3 One approach taken to discuss taboos and stigma about autism in Jamaica's society: 'The experiences of mothers of children with autism in Jamaica: An exploratory study of their journey'.
Autism in the Jamaican society
In *The Chronicles from Jamaica* Maia Chung writes   30

Chapter 4 Inspirational and prominent autistic people around the world.
Caucasian people with autism
People of African descent with autism
Asian people with autism   41

Chapter 5 My journey with autism and my son
From conception to birth
From 21 months to five years old   48

Chapter 6 Boys of African-Caribbean descent overrepresented with a diagnosis of autism in a particular outer London borough   57

Chapter 7 The solution to autism   65

Chapter 8 Autism is not the parents' fault   72

Chapter 9 Let's embrace our beautiful gift   82

Chapter 10 Zeke from birth to 21 months   95

Chapter 11 A continuation of my journey
Excerpts from my home observations   114

Chapter 12 Zeke from diagnosis at age 5 years to 19 years   120

Chapter 13 Picture Exchange Communication (PECS)/
Makaton / Learning Targets and Reports from schools   133

Chapter 14 Lack of support from a Social Worker representative   152

Chapter 15 My career, profession and life postponed   155

Chapter 16 Fears after the diagnosis of autism in my son   161

Chapter 17 Zeke's transition to adulthood   174

Chapter 18 Zeke's educational achievements up to age 19   182

Chapter 19 Photographs of Zeke and his family members   184

Chapter 20 Guidance to Paediatric Health Visitors   189

Chapter 21 Contribution to autistic families   191

Chapter 22 Going on holidays with Zeke   211

Chapter 23 Meltdowns and Zeke's quirky ways   217

Chapter 24 Sample report on Zeke's liability claim   225

Summary   231

Conclusion   233

Glossary of words 245
Appendices: Resources/ References/Blurb 246
Covid Pandemic Anthology Stories 248

INTRODUCTION

'The true measure of a society is how it treats its most vulnerable.' GANDHI

The term 'autism' was a word I came to learn at age 26 in 1984 whilst on a work placement from Brunel University. I was placed at the Education Welfare office in Stoke Newington, north London and was assigned to visit a selection of special schools in Hackney, East London. I can recall visiting about six special schools but one in particular stood out to me.

I observed children in the age group 5 to 16. They looked very normal, yet they seemed restless, moving agitatedly, making lots of different noises and some were banging their heads against the brick walls. Some were biting and lashing out at each other for no obvious reasons. These observations were made during a gymnastic session. At first, I thought that the children needed discipline so I blamed their parents because I believed that they were left to their own devices at home. However, when I spoke to my student supervisor, an educational psychologist, he explained to me that it was the autism condition that caused them to behave the way they were doing. Never, in my wildest dream, did I entertain the thought that one day one of my own children would somehow develop the same autism condition.

In order for me to gain further knowledge of historical theories or facts about autism, I did the following. I investigated how developing countries are meeting the educational needs of autistic children. I also investigated how the general public is being educated in order to remove taboo and prejudice surrounding the autistic child and their parents. To do so, it was necessary for me to research a selection of special schools in Jamaica, the country of my birth. With this new-found knowledge in hand, I was also able to make comparisons between educational provision for autistic children in the borough and country of my current residency, in the United Kingdom. My approach involved reading a selection of newspaper articles, which has been very informative and easy to understand.

CHAPTER 1:
What is autism?

'When you focus on someone's disability you'll overlook their abilities, beauty and uniqueness. Once you learn to accept and love them for who they are, you subconsciously learn to love yourself unconditionally.'
Yvonne Pierre, *The day my soul cried: A memoir*

The autism condition consists of a wide spectrum. It is often described as being on a continuum from 0 to 10. For example.
0_____5_____10
Those children who are assessed as being below 5 on the continuum line usually have speech and are called 'children with Asperger's'. The term 'Asperger's' derives from a famous clinician called Dr Hans Asperger. However, those children who are assessed as being from 5 to 10 are the true 'autistics'. These children range from children with repetitive, disruptive , aggressive behaviours, and single-word speech, to being completely mute or non-verbal. Other conditions connected to the autism spectrum disorder (ASD) include; attention hyperactive disorder (AHD), obsessive compulsive disorder (OCD), Tourette syndrome (TS) and dyspraxia.

Children on the autism spectrum have problems with social communication and interaction, and they may often exhibit certain behaviours which include the following:
- Avoid eye contact
- Are unable to express what they are feeling and thinking through the use of language
- Have a high-pitched or flat voice
- Find it hard to keep up with a conversation
- Have trouble controlling emotions, for example they will hug a stranger
- Lack inhibition - will leave their homes inappropriately dressed, even naked, with bare feet
- Do not take 'no' for an answer
- Use actions to express wants, for example pointing, hitting, biting, scratching, banging their head on the wall, throwing themselves on the floor and screaming
- Use sounds to express wants
- Perform repetitive behaviours such as hand flapping, rocking, jumping, or twirling

Children on the autistic spectrum may repeat certain types of behaviour when it comes to play. They may have a problem with 'make believe' play. They may be more interested in parts of a toy instead of the whole toy. Most of them need strict schedules and often do not like changes to their daily routines. It is exciting to know that some ASD adults live independently on their own and hold down a job. Secondary school children who have had independent travel training can eventually go to school independently. Amongst this group, it is not obvious that they have a condition. Others, on the other hand, have severe disabilities, while many are somewhere between the two ends of the spectrum.

With regard to the cause of autism, scientists believe that genetics is one of the risk factors, although they don't yet have all the answers. The reason is that not just one single gene is involved. There are many factors in addition to genetics.

According to the National Institute of Neurological Disorders in the United States, ASD is characterised by social impairments, communication difficulties, and restricted and repetitive patterns of behaviour. For example, some children with ASD may fail to respond to their names and often avoid eye contact. They have difficulty interpreting what others are thinking or feeling because they cannot understand cues such as tone of voice or facial expressions. They also do not watch other peoples' faces for cues.

In the 1960s it was believed by many people that the cause of autism was due to parents giving their young children hot drinking chocolate mixed with the narcotic *LSD. One of the best known portraits of autism is the 1988 film *Rain Man*. Symptoms of autism vary widely. The word 'autism' was first used in 1910 by Eugen Bleuler, a Swiss psychiatrist. Bleuler described autism as a state in which 'thought is divorced from logic and reality.' Between the 1920s and 1930s, autism was described as a type of childhood schizophrenia.

In 1943 an Austrian psychiatrist, Dr Leo Kanner, described autism as a 'disorder in its own right', but in the 1950s he joined others by agreeing with mother-blaming and stated that autism is due to a lack of maternal warmth to the child. In 1967, in Chicago USA, others were arguing that autism develops due to the 'refrigerator mother'. As a result mothers were encouraged to put their infant in a room with their peers and allow them to do whatever their imaginations (ids), ego, and superegos told them to do. This entire process also involved the mothers undergoing psychoanalysis while the children 'unshackle' themselves with their peers.

The current belief by many people is that the triple jab immunisation injection called the MMR (Measles Mumps and Rubella) is the cause of autism in infants. Views on ethnic background indicate that a lack of vitamin D during pregnancy could point to another cause of autism in the large number of children of African descent who get diagnosed every year. Autism involves a multi-disciplinary field which includes professionals such as biologists, geneticists, psychologists, psychiatrists and pharmacists. Consequently, it should be said that in order to study the mind, it is also necessary to study the brain and the body.

Recent data collected in several countries point to an increase in the number of children being diagnosed with autism.

In response to this increase, the Ministry of Education, through the Education System Transformation Programme (ESTP), has put forward plans to improve the capacity of local educators to better equip them to educate students with ASD.

In regard to this situation in Jamaica, Maureen Samms-Vaughan, Professor of Child Health and Behaviour Development, has confirmed that annually there is a 15% increase in the number of children born with autism. This percentage is equivalent to approximately 500 children and this has created a huge challenge for parents, carers and teachers.

As part of their plan to improve special education provision, the Ministry of Education in Jamaica, through the ESTP, has recently held a three-day training session to equip teachers with greater skills to teach children with ASD . According to Hal Houseworth, a behavioural analyst, over the past five years there has been an increase in the type of information given on autism. As a result of this information more people have become more aware of how best to treat and stimulate people with autism, including children.

In a comparison between boys and girls with autism, the statistics show the ratio of boys to be higher than girls. For every five children diagnosed with autism, four of them will be boys and only one will be a girl. Hence, we have a ratio of 4:1. The age of the father at conception has also proven to be significant. The older the father is at conception, the more likely that his child will develop autism. Therefore, according to the Simon Foundation Autism Research Institute (SFARI), there is a strong belief by researchers in the field of autism that autism is genetic. They have argued that there are up to 400 genes that can cause autism. Ami Qui, a researcher in this field, explained that paediatricians and researchers use lack of eye contact to diagnose ASD.

CHAPTER 2:
The Autism spectrum

Dean Beadle discusses his views and experience of autism
'My future depends mostly upon myself' Paul Robeson

Part A of the diagnostic criteria for Asperger's syndrome focuses on qualitative impairment in social interaction and requires that at least two of four characteristics are to be met in order for the subject to be considered as having social impairment.

The sub criterion mentions a marked impairment in the use of multiple non- verbal behaviours such as lack of eye to eye contact, lack of facial expressions, unusual body postures, and gestures which are needed to regulate social interaction.

Fixations and special interests are other criteria that clinicians and educationalists use to determine if a person is autistic. However, this attribute may be enough to motivate and to prompt an autistic person to engage in social behaviour in order to reach out and communicate.

Autism spectrum disorders (ASD) include social, communication and behavioural challenges. These problems can be mild, severe, or somewhere in between. Therefore, early diagnosis is important, because early treatment can make a difference. Until recently experts talked about different types of autism, such as autistic disorders, Asperger's syndrome and pervasive developmental disorder(PDD), but now all are called (ASD). Asperger's syndrome is at the milder end of the spectrum. A person with Asperger's may be very intelligent and able to handle his or her daily life effectively. They may be very focused on topics that interest them and discuss these tirelessly. They might find it much harder to mix and socialise with others.

The term 'Pervasive Developmental Disorder' (PDD) is no longer used. It is now called and included as Autism Spectrum Disorder (ASD). This diagnosis includes most children whose autism is more severe than Asperger's but not as severe as 'Autistic Disorder'. Autistic disorder is an older term and is further along the autistic spectrum than Asperger's and PDD. It includes the same type of symptoms, but is at a more intense level. Childhood Disintegrative Disorder was the rarest and most severe part of the spectrum. It described children who develop normally and then quickly lose social, language, and mental skills, usually between the ages of 2 and 4. Often, these children will also develop a seizure disorder. Children with Rett syndrome often have behaviours similar to autism, and at one time, experts grouped them among 'ASD'. But now that Rett Syndrome is known to be caused by a genetic mutation, it is no longer considered an autistic disorder.

In order to diagnose and treat, doctors observe the child

and ask the parents a set of questions, mainly about the child's behaviour. At present, there is no known laboratory test for Autism Spectrum Disorder (ASD). The sensible action is to find out as soon as possible if your child is on the spectrum. By doing so, resources can be put in place to help your child achieve their milestones or goals and objectives. Medication is also available to help those children with specific symptoms. However, medication is more effective when used alongside therapy that develops socialisation and other life skills. The best treatment for the ASD child is to appreciate them for who they are, with their unique personalities and their interests, without forgetting to practise the skills which the specialist has introduced to your child.

An example of these unique personalities, talents and interests is demonstrated in Rain Man, the 1988 movie starring Dustin Hoffman and Tom Cruise. In this movie, Hoffman was able to memorise strings of numbers on cards at a gambling table in Las Vegas, USA.

CHAPTER 3:
One approach taken to discuss taboos and stigma about autism in Jamaica's society.

The Experiences of Mothers of Children with Autism in Jamaica: An Exploratory Study of Their Journey.
(Angela R. Mann, University of South Florida, January 2013)
(Google search Angela R. Mann, Email: angelamann@gmail.com)

'There can be no keener revelation of a society's soul than the way in which it treats its children.'   Nelson Mandela

This student research study is not by a trained professional but indicates that some mothers of autistic children believe Jamaican taboos about autism came from 'trimming hair before the child is talking' and 'having a baby out of wedlock'. Further research indicates that these taboos are actually as old as mankind, perhaps derived from Judaism, Buddhism and ancient Mongolia where the cutting of hair is similar to that of 'killing' a person. (Regarding this I searched using taboo hair trimming as an example,). These taboos are also believed in Jamaica and worldwide, and are as old as humanity.

The Mann study uses a lot of quotes from Jamaican mothers, which are written in the dialect. I find this demeaning, but I do understand that to do a quote in a research paper, it does have to be exact.

Wikipedia indicates that Judaism commenced in the 1400s, which by my understanding is untrue. This is the time period when people left Spain, the Middle East and Africa. The African immigration was much earlier, bringing with them ancient rituals and taboos that have been lost with the influx of many different religions. In the following Biblical texts (Ezekiel 5:1-4; Corinthians 1, 11:15, Leviticus 19:27, Numbers 6:5 et al) attending to hair and chastity are seen as holy (good) and not following the Biblical text is seen as unholy (bad). So, perhaps this is where the taboo began. Immigrants to Jamaica did not speak the Jamaican language and these religious texts were translated poorly and caused 'hair trimming' to become forbidden or taboo. I'm from Jamaica and I can see how this might have impacted on the innocent Jamaicans who were deluged with foreigners.

The following is a YouTube video made by a father to help teach people about autism. https://youtu.be/6fy7gUIpMs.

The Jamaican Association on Intellectual Disabilities (JAID) has a mission to provide dynamic leadership, advocacy and influence. This organisation facilitates full integration and inclusion of persons with intellectual disability and other developmental disabilities in society.

In Jamaica, JAID works through education, advocacy and

research to improve the quality of life for families, children and adults who have intellectual disabilities. Their aim is to prevent the causes and the effects of intellectual disability. It is stated that Randolph Lopez did not know much about his daughter Laura's condition of intellectual disability, but he knew he loved her. Therefore, his love for her led him to travel to England where he learned as much as he could about intellectual disability and other disabilities.

At that time there were no facilities in Jamaica well enough equipped to address the special needs of intellectually disabled children. In 1956 when Randolph Lopez returned to Jamaica, he and a core group of parents and friends of children with intellectual disability worked together to set up the first such establishment. Known at that time as 'The School of Hope', it has recently been renamed 'The Schools of Special Education'.

This core group and a number of volunteers then formed 'The Jamaican Association for Mentally Handicapped Children'. This association soon expanded to include adults, and the organisation was re-christened 'The Jamaican Association on Mental Retardation' (JAMR).

In 1974 the Government of Jamaica joined the partnership, and today The Schools of Special Education has a network of 28 schools island-wide. They jointly operate with the Ministry of Education.

In 2004, JAMR celebrated fifty years of advocacy and creating opportunities for people with intellectual disabilities. During this same year JAMR, along with other global entities, signed The Montreal Declaration, a commitment on Intellectual Disabilities. JAMR therefore dedicated itself to the resounding commitment of being part of a global community to address the rights and needs of intellectually disabled people worldwide.

In 2009, JAMR was re-named again as 'The Jamaican Association on Intellectual Disabilities,' (JAID) to reflect the international commitment of The Montreal Declaration. Volunteers, parents and professionals constitute a significant section of JAID's membership. They all share Randolph Lopez's love for special children and work through education. JAID also works closely with the government as well as non-governmental organisations (NGOs).

There appears to be a strong integral training programme led by JAID with both government-funded schools and private fee-paying Jamaican schools. Every effort is being made by this organisation to retain and sustain children with a diagnosis of autism in mainstream schools. The deciding factor, which seems to interfere with children being placed or remaining in special schools, is if they present challenging and unmanageable behaviour for the teacher to handle. When teachers are presented with children who have intellectual disability, JAID's advocacy element has put in place a mentoring programme for those children to learn and develop their full potential alongside mainstream children.

In terms of difficult behaviour, the teacher would also be given strategies and techniques as to how to manage the students' behaviour. The parents or carer would also be involved in these arrangements. It is only when all efforts to integrate the child and to change his or her behaviour have been unsuccessful that the decision is taken to withdraw the child from mainstream school and place them in a special school.

The special schools function as both a day school as well as a residential school. This means that some children are picked up from their home or dropped off each morning and return home each evening. Some children are picked up from the school at the weekend or dropped off by their parents on Sunday evening and sleep over until Friday evening when they return home to their families. There are also holiday projects arranged at the schools where pupils and students engage in activities that are different to what they usually do during term times.

JAID also prides itself on the volunteer programme they have in place. This programme involves volunteers with a range of creative skills to facilitate the programme and teach the students new skills. These skills enable most of the job-seeking students to acquire employment in various external industries. The craft skills include candle making, wooden artefacts and display items, and printing on materials. The students also engage in cooking healthy dinners and baking a variety of cakes and breads for different occasions.

Parents and family members of these students are also encouraged to get involved in their child's school. Parents undergo training to better understand the severity of their children's intellectual disability. Parents are taught how to better stimulate their child and to better manage their unacceptable behaviour. Fathers who are farmers are encouraged to become involved in the school to teach the students their farming skills. Each school has a plot of land specially set aside for farming a wide selection of vegetables such as yams, sweet potatoes, dasheen, coco, chocho, tomatoes, onions, escallion. They learn to plant and reap herbs such as thyme, mints, cerasee. Fathers who are carpenters will usually create bulky play equipment from fallen trees. The children will then be motivated to stand around and watch the process, or even get involved in the making of bulky play equipment, such as climbing frames and see-saws.

Some parents benefit greatly from attending the training programmes that each school has in place for them. These benefits include securing permanent jobs working with the children at the school. These jobs could be classroom teaching assistants or one-to-one support assistants. Some of the parents are given jobs in the residential element of the school. They will work as care assistants, cooks, cleaners and are assigned to other domestic duties.

Despite the good efforts of JAID, there appears to be limitations in the range of resources necessary for the progress and wellbeing of the intellectually disabled children in Jamaica. Maia Chung argues that Jamaica's autism resources for families are meagre. She continues her argument by saying that 'The Jamaican populace isn't really fully educated about autism'. Maia Chung, who is founder of The Maia Chung Autism and Disabilities Foundation (MCADF) 2011, writes, 'When they see a little kid like Quinn acting out, they say that he is spoiled or rude.'

In my opinion, this attitude is not unique to the Jamaican child but is common worldwide. What is needed is a deliberate training program where people who are ignorant of the condition and symptoms of autism get educated in that field. This training is possible, by the mere fact that JAID already provides advocacy to both government-run schools, as well as to independent schools, and Adonijah special schools. Staff, students and parents could be included, amongst all other schools on the island, to receive support and training available from the JAID organisation.

The Adonijah Group of Schools is located in Kingston. It is said to be approved, regulated and monitored by the Jamaican Ministry of Education. It caters for autistic and other children with special needs. Maia Chung described the staff at these schools as excellent.

At Adonijah schools, students with special needs are taught subjects like cooking and Spanish. Maia has reported that her son Quinn is doing outstandingly well and has been found to have 'genius abilities in mathematics'. She has added that the school wishes to enter him for the national maths competition. He has been found to be able to multiply three-digit numbers at a single glance, getting the answer correct each time. Maia emphasised that her son Quinn is in the 'popular group' with his friends.

Maia reiterated that despite limited resources, the model of teaching and interventions at Adonijah have enabled Quinn to be moved into a class with children who do not have special needs. In his class, he is being groomed to take the entrance exam for a regular high school. Maia continued by saying, 'At a recent meeting of similar institutions, the principal of Adonijah reported that Adonijah is currently the only school for 'special needs children' that has had students pass for College High School in Jamaica, which is a traditional high school.' Maia continues that when Quinn was diagnosed with autism, she could never imagine him falling in love, ever getting married and never having a best friend. So far, he's had best friends and someone has already proposed to him on 'Facebook'.

Maia concluded that although Quinn has accomplished many things as a young boy living with autism, she does not know what these accomplishments really mean to someone who has autism. She emphasises that he cannot share these 'highs, lows and excitement' of life with people who love him and those he loves. She questions whether his smiles mean that he's happy. When things bother him, he puts on a sad face, and he cries but is often unable to figure out why he's sad. In these instances she hugs him tight and hopes that he will feel her empathy towards him.

Maia added that eleven years after the birth of Quinn her family founded the MCADF in Jamaica. In 2014 when the foundation was six years old, hundreds of autistic children like Quinn received help. This means that the foundation was formed in 2008.

In the *Autism Chronicles from Jamaica,* Maia Chung writes:

'If you were to conduct an unofficial survey amongst the affected, you would find that autism is a health issue that is minimally addressed by the Jamaican government.' Maia Chung feels that this is a scary and disheartening situation for parents like herself, who formed the client base of the MCADF in April 2008. This client base was formed in response to the very little information and support available for families affected by autism in Jamaica.

She added that as a developing nation, Jamaica's statistics are not always up to date and despite not having a definite prevalence figure in Jamaica, they still have cause for concern. Anecdotal research conducted by the MCADF sees the growth being recorded empirically. Emprical evidence is attained through experience or observation using the five senses. For example a Jamaican born psychiatrist and grandfather of two autistic children stated that when he was a young medical student in the 1970s none were found. 'If the national health records recorded even two cases of diagnosed autism annually it was considered a lot.'

He continues: 'Fast forward three decades later, 2010: There are now hundreds of cases being diagnosed and recorded annually. This fact,' he added, 'is confirmed by the premier authority on autism in Jamaica' who then informed researchers of the Maia Chung Autism and Disabilities Foundation

(MCADF). The opinion amongst health professionals here is that there may be just as many autistic undiagnosed as those who are diagnosed. They concluded that this could be attributable to the complexity of the disorder which has many varied manifestations.

TWO OTHER ESTABLISHMENTS FOR CHILDREN WITH LEARNING DIFFICULTIES IN JAMAICA

The Sure Foundation Educational Centre (SFEC) is a special school which caters for students in the age group 11-21. Their ethos is that every child has the capacity to learn. As a result, they should be given the opportunity to learn. SFEC provides education for children and young people with learning difficulties in a warm and friendly atmosphere by trained and motivated staff. They have three main goals:

1) to provide alternative educational opportunities for children and young people who are unable to cope in mainstream school.
2) To bring students into spiritual awareness of themselves, their potential, their abilities and their responsibilities.
3) To prepare students to meet specific qualifications in order to access further educational opportunities.

Here are two reviews which I believe sum up the credibility of this school.

'The school is making a great impact on the lives of many students.'

'The place my special needs child learned to read and

interact with his peers.'

The second school mentioned above is called Windsor School of Special Education. This school serves students specifically with ASD between the ages of 6-18. This school is also comprised of three campuses in the following areas; May Pen, Spanish Town and Greater Portmore.

CHAPTER 4:
Inspirational and prominent ASD people around the world with some of their favourite quotes.

'Disability is a matter of perception. If you can do just one thing well, you're needed by someone.' Martina Navratilova

Caucasian people with autism

1. Albert Einstein, who died in 1955, had ADHD. He was described as absentminded, a rebel, and a loner. He developed the theory of relativity. "If you can't explain it simply, you don't understand it well enough."
2. Sir Richard Branson, who established the Virgin record deal, has ADHD/dyslexia. "Don't be embarrassed by your failures, learn from them and start again."
3. Michael Phelps - the world's greatest swimmer. "If you want to be the best, you have to do things that other people aren't willing to do."
4. Susan Boyle - a talented Scottish singer who was diagnosed only in 2012. "There are enough people in the world who are going to write you off. You don't need to do that to yourself."

5. Temple Grandin has Asperger's- she brought awareness of autism to the public. "It is never too late to expand the mind of a person on the autism spectrum. There needs to be a lot more emphasis on what a child can do instead of what he cannot do."
6. James Durbin - a talented singer who has Asperger's as well as Tourette syndrome
7. Daryl Hannah – a famous actress
8. Robert Harling-Writer and Producer of a film called 'Steel Magnolias'
9. Dan Aykroyd - He starred in and co-wrote the *Ghostbusters* movie
10. Adam Young -singer
11. Lady Hawke -singer
12. Adam Leven - singer
13. Justin Timberlake - A famous singer who has ADHD
14. Ty Pennington - American television host, former model and actor, artist, carpenter, author, philanthropist - has ADHD.
15. Pete Rose -famous baseball player - has ADHD
16. Howie Mandel - comedian - has ADHD
17. David Newman - a role model of ASD. Owns a successful business and has four airlines. He is also an ADHD motivational speaker.
18. Peter Howson - an artist from Scotland who found comfort in religion.
19. Claire Marzo - a champion Hawaiian surfer.

ASIAN PEOPLE WITH A DIAGNOSIS OF AUTISM
1. Satoshi Zebedia Tajiki - creator of the Pokémon franchise
2. Hikari Oe - pianist - Japanese composer who has autism

PEOPLE OF AFRICAN DESCENT WITH A DIAGNOSIS OF AUTISM
1. Thomas Wiggins was believed to be autistic. He was born blind into slavery in 1849. (It's important to note that slavery was outlawed or abolished in 1833.) He was able to repeat conversations up to ten minutes long, yet he was unable to communicate his wants and needs. He discovered the piano at the tender age of four years and began playing what he heard the daughter of the plantation owner playing. He eventually became a piano player prodigy in that he was able to repeat any piano composition he heard, despite how difficult others found them to play.
2. Paul Robeson and Michael Jackson were in their adult years when they were categorised as having Asperger's Syndrome. "My future depends mostly upon myself" (Paul Robeson).
3. Whoopi Goldberg has been diagnosed as having Attention Deficit Hyperactive Disorder (ADHD). ADHD is common amongst those individuals who are high on the autistic spectrum. "I am where I am because I believe in all possibilities." "Everything for me is visual. That's how my head works." "We're born with success. It is only others who point out our failures, and what they attribute to us as a failure."

4. After viewing a film performed by Paul Robeson in 1947 and a personal interview, Norman Ledgin, a famous clinical psychologist and writer, concluded that Paul Robeson exhibited the non-verbal behaviour of 'reduced eye to eye contact'. Ledgin commented that his take on this matter was that Paul Robeson was slightly impaired in the area of non-verbal expression.

Ledgin went on to say that Paul Robeson's eye contact was not always steady, but was darting in periods when he seemed a bit 'wired' or eager to inform others about little-known phenomena. Ledgin continues by saying that during such periods, Paul Robeson had a tendency to go on about obscure details without recognising the effect that such deliveries were having on listeners.

Even today, the difficulty with eye to eye contact continues to be a hallmark of autism. It has been reported that people with autism and Asperger's have either an inability to make eye contact or a tendency to make too much eye contact to the point of staring. According to Ledgin, Paul Robeson had trouble with the former, i.e. the inability to make eye contact.

Ledgin related that Paul Robeson exhibited a 'loner's temperament' throughout his school years and, as a result, was able to retreat at will to an inner monastic fortress. Ledgin proceeded to add that Paul Robeson's tendency to speak continuously, without recognising cues that the listener was not engaged, indicated a 'lack of social or emotional reciprocity'. In other words, Paul Robeson went on and on about a single subject without being aware that his listeners were tired of hearing about it. Today, the above description of Paul Robeson's speaking behaviour is being observed in other people with Asperger's and seems to be one of the recognisable hallmarks of Asperger's.

It is now widely believed by many that social interaction for adults with Asperger's proves difficult. Paul Robeson has proved this belief inaccurate because he was able to form romantic relationships to the point where he courted and married his wife.

In addition, other people with autism such as Rudy Simone, Liane Holliday-Willey, John Elder Robinson and others have been able to enter into and maintained romantic relationships. "Life is about making a contribution, not about being popular and fitting in." Rudy Simone. "I can only imagine how difficult it must be for someone facing racial or social prejudices to add autism to their list of struggles. It might be less stressful and at times, easier, to ignore the autism. "Lianne Holliday-Willy. "Find your strengths and interests." Learning to get along with other people is vital for our own success and happiness." "Building up a weakness just makes you less disabled. Building a strength can take you to the top of the world." John Elder Robinson

Paul Robeson used his fixations and special interests during the awakening period of the 1930s to engage in social behaviour and reached out and communicated with others. As a result he became more outspoken about civil rights, racial equality, workers' rights and anti-imperialism. Consequently, he gained the admiration and attention of notable figures such as Einstein, Eleanor Roosevelt, Dubois Lena Horne, and Jawaharlal Nehru, the first prime minister of India.

5. The late Michael Jackson, the legendary singer and dancer born in 1959, was diagnosed with Asperger's in 2003, six years before his death. It has been reported that he would watch the same TV footage over and over again. He once had a 'total meltdown' when he had been watching the same James Brown video for four hours and was interrupted.

6. Stephen Wiltshire is a black British architectural artist who was born on 24 April 1974. He is recognised for his ability to draw a landscape from memory after seeing it only once. He received the merit of the Order of the British Empire in 2006 for his contribution to art. At the age of three years he was diagnosed with autism and mutism. "Do the best you can and never stop."

7. Simone Biles, born on 14 March 1997, was diagnosed with ADHD at the age of ten years. Miss Biles was already competing as a level 8 gymnast. She became the first black African-American athlete to win gold in the all-round championship. At the 2016 Olympics in Rio de Janeiro she became the first female US gymnast to win 4 gold medals at a single Games. "I'd rather regret the risk that didn't work out than the chances I didn't take at all. I was built this way for a reason, so I'm going to use it." Simone Biles

This knowledge of the achievements of these people above gives me peace of mind and comfort that there is hope for my son Zeke to achieve success. It is, therefore, my duty and the duty of his educators to identify his gifts and interests, put strategies in place for him to become focused, and to encourage him to develop those identified skills and interests.

CHAPTER 5:
My journey with autism and my son

"I can only imagine how difficult it must be for someone facing racial or social prejudices to add autism to their list of struggles. It might be less stressful and at times, easier, to ignore the autism."   Lianne Holliday-Willey

A POEM FOR MY ASD SON ZEKE
Dear Son
I often wonder is it me,
Is it your dad?
Is it in God's plan that you have autism?
I've explored all possibilities
But have not got a definitive answer
I guess we simply have to plod on together
With what other challenges that life throws at us
In life I promise To be by your side, To offer a helping hand
Whenever you're in need of help
In my departure from this earth
I hope I will have instilled in you
Enough courage and willpower
To face up to life's challenges that devour

FROM CONCEPTION TO BIRTH

I was exactly 39 years old when Zeke was conceived and his father Zephie was 43. For me it was a pleasant surprise, knowing I had experienced the trauma of having a miscarriage 18 months earlier. It was a true blessing for me to know that I was coming to the end of the prime of life and would not like to even entertain the thought of having another baby in my forties. I started to reduce my workload for fear of losing another baby to miscarrying. I immediately reduced my work days as a primary school teacher to two days.

My husband Zephie did not take too kindly to this revelation that I was pregnant.

'Why would you want to go and have another baby? Are you mad?' he squealed. I replied, 'No I'm not mad, darling, but at our age this is going to be my last chance of having another child.'

'Have you considered your medical condition? What advice has the doctor given to you? Will you remain taking the warfarin?' He shook his head in bafflement and left the bedroom. 'I told you I didn't want another child.'

I knew then that I was going to be on my own throughout the pregnancy. But I was determined and happy to be having my last baby who would become my 'washy', a term that is used in my Jamaican culture to describe a woman's last-born child.

We kept the pregnancy quiet between ourselves until five months gestation, when my bump was becoming noticeable.

When I told my secondborn, Cuffie, he was excited. He

remarked 'I been praying for God to give you another child, and my prayer is answered!' When I told our 16-year-old daughter Kelsey, she quietly responded, 'What do you want to go and have another child for? You've already got a girl and a boy.' When I told my older sister Nevaeh her only response was, 'You still do demda sometin?'(those something) with a smile on her face. My older brother Oliver seemed pleased and had a smile on his face. Then he remarked by saying, 'I wish you all the best in your pregnancy.'

The pregnancy was reasonably pleasant, two weeks of mild morning sickness. I had two brief overnight stays in hospital for observation purposes. At twenty-two weeks I started experiencing severe pain and vomiting in the lower right side of my abdomen. This started after having eaten a rotai meal brought to our home by a friend, Deena. I was placed on bed rest for three nights and received medication which got rid of the pain and vomiting. I went home feeling very fit and well but decided that I should not return to my teaching job. My general practitioner (GP) decided to put me forward to receive incapacity benefit.

The second time I was hospitalised, I was thirty-six weeks pregnant. On this occasion the paediatrician was concerned for the baby's position: the head was still not engaged. Anyhow, I was discharged to go home as some babies don't become engaged until the day of birth.

My first option for giving birth was induction and vaginal birth at exactly forty weeks gestation. Elective caesarean with epidural was my second option. I felt it was the safest method for both baby and mother, although deep down I was hoping that it would not get to that.

I was admitted at 10 am on 27 October 1998 to undergo a pre-planned induced labour. After six hours of having the pessaries inserted in my cervix it was evident that labour was not going to start. The medical team were now showing concern, especially since the baby's head was still not engaged. This means that the head is not yet descended into the pelvis ready for the birthing process. My stomach was also starting to feel softer and not as solid as before. One male doctor tried to insert his hand up my vagina to pull the baby down but his hand appeared to be too large to reach my cervix to remove the plug from the cervix to commence the labour.

Despite all the attempts to start the labour, it would not get started. At 3pm it was decided that I should be 'nil by mouth', meaning that I should not eat or drink. A drip consisting of saline solution was inserted into my left arm. It was a painful process getting the needle into my vein, but eventually, after about fifteen minutes, it was successfully in place. At 7am the following day I woke up bright and early and, in anticipation of my baby's caesarean delivery, I decided to have a warm shower. However, I was not aware that a team of doctors were waiting outside my hospital room to commence an emergency caesarean operation.

I only became aware when a young midwife knocked on the shower room door and sternly said, 'Mrs Sailsman! Do you want to give your baby a chance to live? If you do, then the doctors are waiting to commence an emergency operation to save your baby's life!' I instantly said, 'How long have I got?' and she said, 'About ten minutes.' Within three minutes I had put on the theatre gown she had handed to me and was ready to go through the doorway of my room, where I met a team of about ten medics with serious faces and solemn eyes. This same midwife directed me to the operating theatre and helped to make me comfortable on the bed.

The anaesthetist was at the head of the bed, quickly attaching up the various tubes inside my arms and inserting the epidural needle into my spinal cord. Despite working very quickly, he was very gentle. The surgeon was a young Asian lady, and she was waiting patiently to commence the surgery to save the life of my baby. After five minutes I began to feel what seemed like pins and needles in my toes. Then, numbness from my abdomen and below. The surgeon poked my abdomen and asked me if it was painful and I said, 'No.' The senior consultant took a seat beside her and said, 'Let's commence.'

By this time Zephie had not yet arrived. Then a phone call instantly came through, and the nurse said, 'Your sister Nevaeh has just arrived.' I was overjoyed to know that I was being supported by a family member. And, should the worst happen to me, my sister would be there to witness the birth of my son and hopefully become involved in his life as a mother figure. Just as the operation was about to commence, there was a young nurse of African descent who approached me and quietly said to me, 'Have you prayed yet?' I solemnly nodded my head and said, 'Yes I have.' At that instance the senior surgeon and the junior surgeon's eyes met and both nodded their head to each other. The junior surgeon started to cut through the muscles of my lower abdomen. At this point, all I could feel was poking, probing and pressure on my abdomen.

The junior surgeon was completely focused on my abdomen while the senior surgeon sitting beside her was watching my face and observing the work of the junior surgeon. All other staff present remained as quiet as a mischief of mice in a state of total observation of both me and the action of the junior surgeon. The anaesthetist was the only person who uttered words; he was quite playful and chatty with me as if using a distraction technique on me for my benefit. My sister Nevaeh was sitting closest to me on my left side. She held my hand in such an unbelievably caring manner. Never in our lifetime together had she had the opportunity to be so gentle and kind to me. But I felt loved, appreciated and respected by her.

Finally, after about ten minutes of cutting through my abdomen, my baby was lifted out of my abdomen. At first he didn't cry, but after one of the doctors took him and cleared mucus from his throat and planted a couple of gentle slaps on his bottom, he gave out three loud cries. He was then shown to me and placed in the arms of my sister Nevaeh while the junior surgeon commenced the process of stitching up my opened abdomen. The anaesthetist adjusted the level of oxygen getting into my system because at that point I said I felt dizzy.

The stitching and suturing took about forty- five minutes until I was ready to return to my individual hospital room. Before I was wheeled back to my room, I was given my baby to hold for the first time. I kissed him and said, 'Hello, baby. You're in the arms of your mummy.' I told him that he was gorgeous. He stared me in the eyes and looked around at everyone else. It was a relief to know that we were both ok. I was looking forward to returning home to commence life with 'God's new gift to the family' and to pick up the pieces with Kelsey, Cuffie, and hubby Zephie.

Zephie did not arrive at my bedside until two hours after Zeke was born. By that time, I was back in my room, and Nevaeh was sitting with me and holding her nephew. As soon as Zephie entered the room, he walked over to me as I lay on my bed, drifting in and out of a deep sleep. He kissed me on the lips and said, 'How you feeling?' and I replied, 'Tired and sleepy.' I then closed my eyes and drifted off to sleep. Zephie went over to where Nevaeh was sitting and holding her nephew. Zephie greeted her and stretched his hand out to hold his baby son for the first time.

After what seemed like one hour, I awoke from my deep sleep and noticed that Zephie was sitting beside Nevaeh holding the baby. Nevaeh was filling him in about the whole process of the caesarean as the baby slept in his arms. Not long after, Nevaeh said she had to leave to go and break the good exciting news to the other children. Zephie remained with me until visiting time was ended at 8pm. He placed the baby on my tummy, kissed me, and said he would be bringing Kelsey and Cuffie to visit us the following day at 3pm. Both children were very excited and pleased to meet their new baby brother. The next day, Cuffie had a short hold of the baby while Kelsey spent most of the time sitting down holding her baby brother carefully in her arms.

Twenty- four hours later the paediatrician surgeon who delivered Zeke by caesarean section entered my hospital room and had a little talk with me about the reason why baby Zeke could not be born normally. She explained that he was a victim of a 'true knot' of the umbilical cord. That term was unknown to me so I asked her to explain. She proceeded to say that the umbilical cord was wrapped tightly around Zeke's neck and that it had a very tight knot in it. She further explained that it would have been impossible for Zeke's head to fit properly into my pelvis since there was not enough length in the umbilical cord due to the knot in the cord and it being so tightly wrapped around his neck. This situation would have made it impossible for me to give birth vaginally. The consequences of such an attempt would have been detrimental to mine and my baby's life.

I was shocked to hear this feedback because my final scan at 38 weeks should have detected such a problem. When I asked the doctor if there was a likelihood that my baby is brain-damaged she said he should be fine because lots of babies each year are born under such circumstances. Most have shown no signs of brain damage and have grown up to become very academic, and others are holding down good jobs and raising families.

Five days later, I talked to one of the midwives who had cared for me during my initial admission on the prenatal ward. I asked her if my baby will be ok. She said he looked fine at the moment but that it's early days for anyone to say. She added that, 'We'll have to wait and see.'

Six weeks later, when I returned to the hospital for my postnatal check-up. I asked the paediatric consultant if my baby is ok, considering the 'true knot' and the umbilical cord so tightly tied around his neck. She looked at me with a serious face and said, 'Look at that baby. No one could say that baby has anything wrong with him. He's fine, he's a healthy baby.'

My baby and I, however, remained in hospital for five days due to concerns about the clotting time of my INR level. Zephie, Kelsey and Cuffie paid daily visits to see us in hospital and after Sunday church one day our pastor and most of the church members showed up at the hospital ward to visit me and the baby. Pastor and one female member took turns holding the baby in the foyer of the ward as the ward sister was resentful of so many people entering the ward at the same time. I had daily visits from Zephie and my older children. It was so exciting when the consultant finally discharged us from hospital. The following day Zephie brought Kelsey and Cuffie along with him to collect baby and me from the hospital. Soon we were all in the car making our way to Enfield for the thirty-minutes' drive. I thank God for everything and for bringing us all safely home.

CHAPTER 6:
Boys of African-Caribbean descent over-represented with a diagnosis of autism in a particular outer London borough.

'If the world thinks you're not good enough, it's a lie, you know that. Get a second opinion.' Nick Vujicic

It has become common talk amongst my acquaintances and me that noticeably a larger number of black boys than boys from other ethnic groups were being diagnosed with severe autism. I'm deeply concerned about this statistic. I and some other black mums would frequently question ourselves in regards to why it is always the reception age black boys whose heads seem to be popping up at the window and looking outside the classroom window while the other children are busy completing their work. We were deeply concerned but could never work out the reasons why that was so. However, for me, having had a son who has had a diagnosis of autism, I will now be able to offer some explanation about why black boys exhibit that specific behaviour.

It's a known fact that teachers enjoy teaching motivated

and well-behaved children. Therefore, children who would be seen as unmotivated and lacking interest would be left to play freely within the classroom. In their idleness, they would disrupt or damage more motivated children's work. The result of this action would cause the teacher to attempt to speak to them about their behaviour and acceptable discipline would be imposed. Parents would be notified, but this unacceptable behaviour would continue. Consequently, plans would be put in place to have this disruptive black boy's behaviour assessed by a psychologist, and consequently he would be given a statement of special needs currently known as an Education Health and Care Plan.

In theory, this youngster would now be eligible for a support worker to assist him to access the curriculum more smoothly within the mainstream classroom. In practice, two things happen: first, the funding money which comes from central government is usually used to fund music and extra-curricular activities for more able students; and secondly, the assigned support worker is frequently withdrawn from the student to engage in other activities around the school. Or, they are often used as interpreters for non-English speaking parents of other children. Hence the student who has been diagnosed with autism is left to his own devices. They would then spend most of this time getting into the way of more able students who would be raising complaints to parents and staff.

Ultimately, the process would commence whereby the ASD student is transferred to a specialist provision which doesn't necessarily meet their educational needs. In extreme cases, most of them will experience abuse of various forms. They generally regress, become withdrawn and unmanageable, and are ultimately placed in sheltered accommodation when they become young adults at 18 years of age.

With this information at my disposal, I proceeded to explore how these findings would compare to schools in Jamaica. My findings were surprising. In Jamaica, I found that the amount of girls diagnosed were similar in number to that of boys. I also found that in Jamaica a greater percentage of youngsters with autism and Asperger's are more likely to proceed to further educational training, although employers are reluctant to offer them permanent jobs. Unfortunately, I was unable to confirm that a greater percentage of autistic Jamaican youngsters were able to hold down jobs, live independently, and have mainstream friends than those living in London.

After reading an article written in the Gleaner by Mr BB who was assigned to the Rural Services for Children with Disabilities in Santa Cruz, St. Elizabeth, Jamaica. I requested an appointment to visit the school with the assistance of Mr BB. The date was set for Friday 3rd November 2017 at 10am. Upon arrival at the school I was met by Miss EK, the Unit Supervisor attached to the school.

Through a conversation with Miss EK I learnt that the Learning Centre is under the umbrella of Woodlawn School of Special Education. Woodlawn School is based in Mandeville and has an efficient and passionate principal. The Santa Cruz

Learning Centre consisted of 31 students with a diagnosis of Learning Challenges. Of the 31 students, 10 are autistic. The age range of the students is seven to eighteen. Resources at Santa Cruz are limited to one I-Pad, and staff demonstrate their imagination and creativity by making resources for the students to work with. There are no speech and language therapists at the Centre. Amongst the students who have ASD, one student has no speech; 4 students have some speech; 5 students have good speech and of this number, 1 of these students has a robotic speech pattern.

Staff receive updated knowledge through a strict termly staff training session. All teaching staff have a Bachelor's Degree in Special Education. All learning support staff have an Early Childhood Education qualification.

In terms of financial support given by the government to parents of autistic children, this is unheard of by staff. Neither are any autistic graduates, so far entered into paid or voluntary, non-paid employment to date. In the past, job applications for the most able students with autism or Asperger's have been submitted to departmental stores but they don't get offered employment.

No young autistic adults from this unit have proceeded to independent living or supported living in residential homes. The trend is that they remain living at home with their parents or with other family members in the event of the loss of the parents or main caregiver. It is unheard of for autistic adults to get married or even have children.

When I asked how I might support the unit, Miss EK suggested that resources are greatly needed within the unit. She would like me to purchase the resources and present them to the unit in person. I have decided to supply 10 iPads to the unit and a few sensory resources that will teach phonics, reading and numbers.

Miss EK continued by saying that integration into mainstream is encouraged and that this arrangement is the preferred channel of education by parents. She added that the result of this decision is that children are called derogatory names, such as 'dummy', by some of the youngsters in mainstream education.

My response to this argument is that name calling is a common practice by most youngsters in mainstream education, particularly when the difficulties are obvious. A stammering but academically gifted peer will at times be called 'ram-goat' or even 'dummy.'

To date there has been a study of 27 nationwide companies that are employing people with autism and Asperger's. Specifically, in England we have an organisation called the National Autistic Society that developed the Voice Magazine which is used widely by families living in the London boroughs.

The German company 'Vodafone' is known for being influential in the usage of codes in the making of mobile phones. This company is widespread in England and has a reputation for employing young people with autism and Asperger's. Vodaphone is also actively training up their managers and business leaders in how to communicate with people with autism and Asperger's. Vodaphone will now employ these people who have the ability to carry out tasks concerning patterns and numbers.

Another company, known as Auticon, believes that autistic people have an eye for detail and a proven power of observation with concentration specifically on the tasks in hand. They have orthographic memory, lateral thinking, loyalty and truthfulness. Regarding orthographic memory, this means, some people who have ASD are able to look at letters and words on the page and then use their knowledge of sound/symbol relationships to sound out tricky words. Regarding lateral thinking, this means, they are able to solve problems using creativity and reasoning that is not immediately obvious to non ASD subjects.

At Ford Automobile Company, especially in the vehicle evaluation and verification laboratory, it is proven that inclusion works. In this department, employees log and prep tyres for test vehicles used by engineers for product assessment. This work is regarded as highly structured, requires a great deal of focus, and calls for a high level of attention to detail and organisation. Ford confirms that these skills are typically associated with individuals with autism. Ford has announced that they have job training programmes for people with autism.

Spectrum Designs USA, a non-profit organisation who do printing on clothes and on other products, also employs people with autism.

A North Carolina non-profit organisation also employs people with autism to do a range of jobs. These jobs include event set-up, laundry service and delivery, data entry, packaging, mailing, dog walking, cat sitting, city bus clean-up and football parking.

An organisation called 'Autonomy Works' creates jobs for people with autism to utilise their analytical talents. Generally speaking we utilise analytical talents when we detect patterns, do brainstorming, observing and when interpreting new data.

'Specialisterne Foundation' has a new approach to hiring autistic people. For example they do Information Technology (IT) services such as software testing, data registration, quality control and information packaging for a number of leading IT and communications companies around the world.

'Technology Start-up Ultra' has jobs for people who have autism in their software testing services.

'Microsoft' has also partnered with the 'Specialisterne' organisation to provide employment for people with autism.

'Amazon' has been recruiting people with autism for employment in their Robots and Computer Departments, specifically for logging algorithms.

'Sordex Company' is a Sardinian company which deals with virtual currency, whereby people exchange with goods and professional services rather than with real money. This company is one of the newest companies with plans to go global and provide employment for people with autism.

The percentage of different biological races that are

employed in the above-mentioned organisations has not been specified. I assume that a fair percentage of people with ASD who are of African origin living in outer London boroughs would also be represented in these work forces that was mentioned earlier. In the local outer London neighbourhood in which I'm based, I have observed people with ASD from families of African origin working in restaurants, takeaway food businesses, coffee shops and car washes.

CHAPTER 7:
The solution to autism

'The only disability in life is a bad attitude.'   Scott Hamilton

Parents and caregivers of children should be vigilant and ensure that from birth babies are cuddled frequently, encouraged to follow eye-hand coordination from the caregiver, observe mouth and tongue movement and copy mouth movements and noises as much as possible. The carer should encourage the baby to learn names of the family as well as single words such as animal names and names of feeding equipment. The main caregiver should make it a routine to read age-appropriate books to the baby, getting them to repeat names of characters in the story as well as sounds made by those characters in the story. Catch phrases are very useful in stories for young babies, which they should be encouraged to learn and repeat.

When all these are in place as a routine, then it makes it easier for parents and caregivers to observe a change or absence of developmental behaviour and speech in their babies.

The parent or caregiver must not hesitate to book an appointment with the health visitor and general practitioner if any changes or absence of behaviour or speech is observed.

Your baby will need an urgent appointment to be assessed by an experienced paediatrician.

The current trend involves a team called the Triage. The Triage Team includes a paediatrician, speech and language therapist, (SLT) and Ears Nose and Throat specialist (ENT). The paediatrician will have specific blood tests done to rule out other conditions such as a condition called Fragile X syndrome.

Fragile X syndrome (FXS) runs in families. Being an inherited condition, FXS can be passed on to the next generation. It is a known cause of a lack of intellectual development. The symptoms of FXS include the following:
- Walking, talking or toilet training much later than other children of the same age
- Trouble making eye contact
- Frequent ear infections
- Trouble sleeping
- Seizures
- Sensory difficulties which involve trouble with what they see, hear, smell, taste and touch.

There is presently no cure for FXS. However, early diagnosis helps families get early treatment and services for their child. The known cause of FXS is due to a change in the genetic material in each cell of the body. A change in this genetic material makes it difficult for cells to produce a certain protein that is necessary for normal brain development and function.

In the assessment to determine if a child has autism, the ENT team will carry out tests to rule out deafness or hearing loss. The SLT will carry out a series of cognitive tests that include following instructions and completing required tasks. These tests ensure how well the baby understands instructions.

I'm a firm believer that babies and toddlers are best cared for by their mothers. Most mothers are natural speakers and have the natural ability to engage in baby talk with their young ones. Most fathers have not got that natural ability, so they're not a natural option for stimulating early speech in babies and toddlers. It's understandable after a busy and tiring day in the work place. Most parents haven't got the energy to speak and interact adequately with these babies and toddlers. But this is a must. Your baby's speech development is dependent on the quality of verbal stimulation that their mothers give to them.

Regardless of how well the caregiver appears to be interacting with their young ones, its imperative and a duty that mothers and caregivers must find time to build up their energy to speak with and interact with their young ones. Bowlby in his attachment theory in 1973 speaks about the effect of 'maternal deprivation' on the young child. It's an absolute must that mothers, especially, spend quality time with their young ones, get down to their level, engage in baby talk with them, play turn-taking games with them and, most importantly, curl up beside them, give them cuddles, kisses and read a bedtime story to them every night.

The Swiss developmental psychologist Jean Piaget in 1936 describes the different stages in a child's development when it's a must that certain skills are developed. He stresses the sensory and motor sensory stages.

For the benefit of my topic on autism, I will focus on the stages for the age groups 0-2 years and 2-7 years because it is usually by the age of 7 that a specialist in the diagnosis of autism can confidently confirm that a child has Autistic Spectrum Disorder. Bowlby, another developmental psychologist, explains that at 0-2 years old the baby coordinates his senses with motor responses. For example, the child will show sensory curiosity about the world. He is interested in the language used for command and cataloguing. He thinks that objects remain static and do not move.

Bowlby continued to explain that at the age of 2-7 the toddler begins to show signs of symbolic thinking. They are able to use proper syntax and grammar to express full concepts. They demonstrate strong imagination and intuition, but their abstract thought is still under-developed. However, their conversation ability is developed. Piaget was the first psychologist to make a systematic study of cognitive development. Piaget showed that young children think in strikingly different ways compared to adults.

Sigmund Freud, 1856-1939, describes phases of a child psychosexual development such as oral, anal, phallic, latency and genital stages. In Freud's view, each of these stages focused on sexual activity and the pleasure received from a particular area of the body. For example in the oral phase, children are focused on the pleasures that they receive from sucking and biting with their mouth, while in the anal phase this focus shifts to the anus as they begin to receive toilet training and the attempt to control their bowel movement.

In the phallic stage, Freud believes that the focus moves to genital stimulation and the sexual identification that comes with having a penis. During this stage Freud thought that children turn their interest and love towards their parent of the opposite sex and begin to strongly resent the parent of the same sex. He called this idea 'Oedipus complex' as it closely mirrored the events of an ancient Greek tragic play in which a king named Oedipus manages to marry his mother and kills his father.

The phallic/Oedipus stage was thought to be followed by a period of latency during which sexual urges and interest were temporarily non-existent. Finally, children were thought to enter and remain in a final genital stage in which adult sexual interests and activities come to dominate. By today's standards, Freud's psycho-sexual theory does not stand and is considered to be inaccurate. However, in my view, the ASD child may at times confirm some of Freud's explanation, particularly his argument for his oral, anal and phallic stages.

SOCIOCULTURAL PERSPECTIVE: VYGOTSKY'S THEORY:

Vygotsky (1896-1934) argues that children are products of their culture. Therefore, children's cognitive development is not only brought about by social interaction, but it is inseparable from the cultural contexts in which children live.

Vygotsky viewed development as an apprenticeship in which children progress by interacting with other children who share understanding among each other in an activity. Cognitive growth results from children's involvement in structured activities with others who are more skilled than they.

For some children these stages are developed naturally. However for others they will need help and encouragement to do so. For that reason, parents need to be encouraging their young ones to achieve these skills. Therefore, parents need to be vigilant in their observation of how their young ones are playing and, if necessary, introduce them to play in age-appropriate ways. For example, babies under two months should be encouraged to put fingers and hand in their mouths or even to be given a dummy or pacifier to suck on.

These actions exercise nerves and muscles in the mouth in preparation for making sounds and talking. It is also beneficial to the baby when mothers practise making sounds with their mouths and encourage their babies to copy these sounds, and mouth and tongue movements.

Mothers should verbalise the word for the object that the baby is pointing to. For example, if the child is pointing to the bottle then the mother should say 'bottle'. Eventually, the mother could add 'Bottle, please' or 'I want bottle.'

At six months old the baby will begin to show interest in anal activities. Therefore, the mother should give them the correct names for activities involving the anus. For example, pooh, wee-wee or urine, potty, toilet, wash hands, sink, toilet paper, soap, nappy, pants etc.

Current guidance from a range of educationalists and psychologists recommends that as soon as an individual child is diagnosed with autism, their parents should seek out diagnostics for the areas in which they are struggling. Various interventions such as applied behavioural analysis, occupational therapy, play therapy, speech and language therapy, athletic therapy and many more have proven to show a positive impact on ASD individuals in these treatments.

After watching the videos involving Dean Beadle, Luke Dicker and Temple Grandin, I have hope that my son Zeke could have a career with a bright future if given opportunities.

CHAPTER 8:
Autism is not your fault

"We're born with success. It is only others who point out our failures, and what they attribute to us as failure"
Whoopi Goldberg

Connie Hammer, a modern theorist, parent educator, consultant and coach, guides parents of young children who have been recently diagnosed with autism spectrum disorder. She helps parents to discover their child's abilities and add possibilities. In an article listed in 'Self Growth.com,' Ms Hammer writes that autism is not the parents' fault. She tells parents that they should not revert to feeling guilty but should instead address their feelings and not allow them to fester. (https:www.selfgrowth.com/articles/my-child-s-autism-is-not-my-fault).

After reflecting on the level of care that my husband, Zeke's older sister, his older brother and I have provided to Zeke, I'm now confident in saying that his autism is not our fault. During my pregnancy, I did not have any accidents or falls, I ate and drank healthily. I also rested well, took mild exercise such as going swimming and going for daily leisurely walks.

From birth we interacted well with Zeke by getting down to his level in different ways.

On the other hand, in the back of my mind, I quietly blamed myself for my son's autism. After all, giving consideration to John Bowlby's (https://en.wikipedia.org/wiki/Maternal deprivation) teaching on the consequences of maternal deprivation, I asked myself the question, 'How could I be so certain that people l hardly know would treat my baby with love, kindness, and empathy to the same extent that I do? How could I be certain that a carer would give my baby the correct type of sensory experience?'

I reflect on Jean Piaget's outlined stages of development. (https://www.learning-theories.com/piagets-stage-theory-of-cognitive-development.html) I remember that Zeke found his feet and was walking by 11 months old. How could I be certain that if my child had a fall his carer would take him to the hospital for a check-up, or even inform his parents? Lastly, and most importantly, how could I be certain that the carer of my child would not entrust my baby to the care of their friends who have criminal intent towards young children? The guilt feelings go on and on. To console myself, I say only God knows, and he will punish my child's carer and all people according to their deeds.

When Zeke was small, I would frequently hold him on my lap and happily talk to him. He would react by blowing bubbles and make sounds whilst making good eye contact with me. I would sing nursery rhymes to him and sometimes when I stopped singing to him he would start crying, and when I resumed singing he would stop crying, smile, and maintain good eye contact with me. He basically talked with his eyes. When he was tired, I would hold him in my arms and gently rock him to sleep. When he was sound asleep I would carefully place him in his Moses basket in the living room downstairs, so that he was never left alone in a room upstairs during the day. If I was tired and needed a nap, I would rest on the sofa which was close beside him. He would be awake for two hours and then sleep for two hours.

Zeke was breast-fed for four months, so during the night time, 'feeding time' was easy and relaxed. When he awoke and as soon as he made a few sounds or would cry, I would pick him up and say something nice to him, kiss him, and then bring him into the bed with us. I would prop my pillows up, make myself comfortable and commence breast feeding him.

He loved to be breast-fed; he would suckle for fifteen minutes, taking short breaks in sucking, and when he had stopped sucking I would lay him on a towel on our bed and commence changing his wet or soiled nappy. After a few minutes, stroking , kissing his cheeks I would talk to him. After which he would fall asleep for about two hours. The same feeding, awakening routine was repeated every night for about three months. At three months he was sleeping twice as long and would remain awake for just as long.

When Zeke was six months old, I developed an appendicitis infection and was hospitalised for three weeks. The emergency situation meant that Zeke had to be in the care of his two mature female cousins, Kay and Trish, with his older sister and brother in their home. When the doctor received all of my blood tests results, it was first decided that I needed an operation to have the appendix removed. Firstly, it was necessary for me to have the appendix drained of all the infection. As a result, my sister Nevaeh decided it was a better idea that all three children, including six-month-old Zeke, should move temporarily to her home from outer London to Islington. Those three days of absence from my baby proved unbearable for me.

What made the situation worse for me was that I was in the middle of planning Zeke's christening, which was scheduled to take place on the fourth day of me being hospitalised. I really did not want to undergo an operation without my baby being christened or blessed. My assigned doctor at the hospital was aware of this, so she tried to persuade me to cancel the christening and plan it again for after I've had my surgery and was fit and well enough to enjoy the occasion.

It was an unfortunate situation that when Zeke was only six weeks old his father and I had a disagreement and we decided that it was best for him to move out of the family home to allow us both time to think things through and then make a final decision regarding our marriage. Although I remained 'nil by mouth', meaning I was not allowed to eat or drink, it was agreed by my consultant that I could be present at my baby's christening.

After the church service, I remained at home with my

guests while they enjoyed the lovely food and drinks that my sister Nevaeh and cousin-in-law Bloss had prepared for them. During this time, I held Zeke comfortably in my arms. He slept most of the time and did not appear to be his usually happy and chatty self. I felt he was missing me, and that made me feel very sad.

I so wished I didn't have to return to the hospital that same evening. My cousin Brenda, her daughter Sophia and another younger cousin, Evelyn, came down from Birmingham to attend the christening. Brenda is one of Zeke's godmothers. They also had to leave to return to Birmingham after the christening party. My niece Trish and cousin Kay happily volunteered to remain at my home to take care of Zeke under the watchful eyes of older sister Kelsy and older brother Cuffie.

I was driven back to the hospital at 8pm by Kelsey's best friend Sheryl's mother, Mary. After being dropped off at the hospital I went into the bathroom to freshen up. I felt extremely tired, so I quickly changed into my night clothes and retired to my bed. However, I observed that the saline needle that was inserted into my arm for easy set-up of my saline drip had pulled out of my arm. I instantly pressed the buzzer to report this to the nurse. I was hopeful that she would put it back in place and attach it again to the saline, since I had not eaten or drunk any fluid since the previous night.

Instead of kindly and sympathetically fixing the problem, the agency nurse began accusing me of pulling out the needle from my vein. 'I see you've pulled out the needle from your arm,' she remarked in a stern voice. I calmly tried to explain that it was accidently pulled when I was changing into my night clothes. She walked away from my bedside in disgust with anger on her face. I then waited until about 11pm, a full three hours since I had initially asked the nurse for help.

In the meantime, I had been speaking with an Indian lady in the next bed beside me. She told me right off that 'I should not allow them to operate on me in this hospital because they had a poor reputation for operations results'. Unfortunately, this hospital was C F in Enfield. As I was already not comfortable having an operation to remove my appendix, I had a thought. That thought was to quickly and discretely get 'redressed' and promptly leave the hospital. In a flash I was dressed and, in no time at all, I was half way down the corridor, making my way to the hospital exit. Another patient in the bed opposite mine realised what my intentions were, so she remarked to me, 'Aren't you going to tell her that you're leaving?' I simply looked at her and did not answer her question. I knew if I told any nurse I was leaving the hospital, they would have attempted to stop me.

Luckily, l knew the location of the taxi station, so I made my way out of the hospital. One small, petite, middle-aged Caucasian nurse attempted to restrict me from leaving, but I told her, 'Don't put your hand on me!' in a stern voice. I also told her if she touched me, I would knock her out flat. Luckily, that scared her off, and I walked out the doorway of the hospital building without looking behind me. The first thing

I knew, I was sitting in the front seat of a people carrier being driven home by a friendly and cooperative Greek male driver. When I arrived home Trish, Kay and Kelsey were shocked. They told me that they had just come off the telephone with a nurse from the hospital. The nurse had told them to expect me to come home anytime now became I had discharged myself from the hospital without permission.

Shortly after I had arrived home, cousin-in-law Bloss rang the house phone. I explained to her the reason why I had discharged myself from the hospital. I also told her that I was concerned about Zeke's wellbeing and how he was missing me and looking ill and withdrawn. Bloss suggested that I should allow her son Marc to drive Zeke and me straight to the Royal Free Hospital's Accident and Emergency which I did. After waiting with severe abdominal pain for about two hours, I passed out and the staff then decided to quickly attend to me. I was then given a bed to lie on, and a cot was brought down for Zeke and placed right beside my bed in a cubicle right there in Accident and Emergency.

A student nurse was assigned to care for Zeke. After a while I was asked to go to rest and sleep because I was looking very tired and stressed. Eventually, a few hours later, we were taken to the postnatal ward where Zeke and I had been placed shortly after he was born. I felt pampered because we were placed into a room by ourselves. I felt happy having my baby with me, and I noticed that Zeke appeared happier and began to make his usual good eye contact with me. He was becoming quite chatty as he had been three weeks previously, before I had developed symptoms of appendicitis and was admitted to hospital.

I was, however, quite disturbed when my sister Nevaeh described Zeke's behaviour and reaction while he was in her care for the two days before Zeke and I were both readmitted to the Royal Free Hospital. She said that he constantly wanted his bottle of milk and that as soon as he had finished drinking, he would burp and break wind from below and produce a heavily soiled nappy. As a result, his nappy had to be constantly changed. Shortly after Nevaeh and her friend, Petra, left the hospital, I noticed that Zeke's naked body was covered with red blotches. It looked like a skin rash typical of an allergic reaction.

I also became concerned that in three hours of being reunited with me, he had produced four heavily soiled nappies after drinking a 7-ounce bottle of milk. I did wonder if these symptoms were evidence of meningitis, so I asked a staff nurse if it was at all possible for my baby to be examined by a paediatrician. To my surprise, after promising that she would look into it for me, she returned two hours later and explained that I was admitted for 'care for myself and not my baby'. Therefore, she was not able to make that request, my request was denied.

I was disappointed with that outcome but decided not to kick up a fuss, as I was still feeling very ill with the appendix infection. I then decided to change the type of powdered milk he was put on for one much milder and the diarrhoea eased.

I also started using baby powder all over his body and within two days the rash cleared up. I concluded that both conditions were due to the type of milk he was being given. Prior to my admission to CFH, he was being breast fed and he did not have the problems I described above. I was discharged from Royal Free hospital after three weeks as an in-patient.

During my stay in hospital, my husband Zephie was still living at home with his mother while Kelsey and Cuffie were staying at my sister Nevaeh's home in Islington. Zephie did visit the hospital twice to see his son and me. I was adamant that it was not necessary for me to have an appendectomy operation unless it was absolutely necessary to do so, since all operations carry a risk of fatality. I was glad when my consultant said that he was going to discharge me with medication and that he would do a follow-up review in three months' time. The following day, after three weeks in hospital, Zephie arrived to pick Zeke and me up from hospital to take us home.

It was a week day, so Kelsey and Cuffie were in school. By now, they had returned home because Zephie had returned home to take care of them. It was such a lovely feeling knowing that I was no longer in pain and that my three children were safe and well. Regarding Zephie and our marital situation, Zephie had suggested that we should work harder at our marriage. It wasn't going to be as straight forward as that, since Zephie still needed to give me some answers to my questions regarding what he had done with the money in our joint savings account.

I wanted to know what he was doing with his income as he was constantly broke and not saving any money even though I had a part-time income coming in and my maternity payment. After a short while I decided to postpone any conversation with Zephie about his mismanagement of his money but somehow we did not have further separation or a divorce.

It's important to note that Zephie has never really blamed me or himself for our son's autism. However he did comment once, when Zeke was about ten years old and his behaviour had become more challenging, that 'Look what you have put yourself through.'

CHAPTER 9:
Embracing your beautiful gift

'Life is not measured by the number of breaths we take, but by the moments that take our breath away.' Maya Angelou

Fast forward, sixteen years. Zeke has been one of the most amazing children I have even known. Despite his quirky ways and his occasional meltdowns, he is loving, kind, sympathetic and considerate. In terms of personality, Zeke loves to be around people, especially those who are considerate to his needs and to his feelings. He enjoys going to our church and he will sit and listen for 75% of the time in church on a Sunday morning.

When he gets agitated and inappropriately quite chatty to his parents as we sit beside him, he is usually cooperative when told to go and join his buddy Elton or Immanuel at the back of the church. He would sit with this buddy for thirty minutes and copy a given scripture from the bible into his note book and draw pictures then colour them-in. At the end of the service, he would join others to have a biscuit or cake before leaving to go home.

Zeke has a tremendous level of kindness. He is always

willing to share his food and drink with others without making a fuss or being scornful. He will carefully and gently hold his three-year-old niece's hand and walk along the pavement slowly and cautiously. As they both walk along the road they are being carefully watched by his parents, meaning Zephie and I, walking slowly behind them.

Zeke demonstrates a huge level of helpfulness. At home his parents can rely on him to follow instructions, such as collecting things they need but are too tired to go and fetch for themselves. He will unpack the dishwasher and stack it with dirty utensils. He will also set the table, as well as clear the table after meals, without being asked to do so.

In terms of independent living skills Zeke routinely bathes, showers and washes himself twice a day without prompting from anyone. He knows how to use the washing machine, including how much detergent and conditioner to put in the various compartments. Zeke is often considerate to the feelings of others and gets upset when younger children are crying and are upset. He will try to offer comfort by offering a piece of tissue and by saying, 'Don't cry.' At home he will set the bath for me even when he hasn't been asked to do so. He is particularly considerate to my needs, his mother. He frequently asks me if I 'want a cup of tea', and when I reply 'Yes please!' he proceeds to the kitchen and makes a lovely cup of tea for me. Zeke is friendly and sociable. He loves to be in the company of youngsters in his age group. He will sit and listen quietly as his peers in mainstream education talk around him, even when they get noisy. He loves to sing, dance and listen to a wide selection of music.

Zeke's passions are computers, sports, athletics, music, singing, dance, drama and art. As a result, our plan for him is that at the age of 19 + he will be transferred to another college where he will study the above-mentioned subjects for three years.

ZEKE'S MOST DISTURBING BEHAVIOURS
From age 3 years and 9 months, Zeke went through a phase of plastering himself all over with his own faeces. This behaviour usually happened after a refreshing bath and having his hair shampooed. When I was overwhelmed by this situation, his father Zephie would calmly give him another bath, strip his bedding and clean the faeces from surfaces in his room.

Whilst attending an educational 'playgroup' staff reported that Zeke would '…take the children's snacks and pile them onto his plate, even though he doesn't eat it.' Whilst attending a local primary school Reception class, it was reported that he kept following a particular little girl around. This little girl did not like him following her around. When she told her mother, her mother told Zeke off in front of me. When I intervened to explain that Zeke does not have speech, she reacted by saying her daughter 'does not like it so he should stop doing it.'

Due to dissatisfaction with our local primary school Zeke was moved to Bowes Primary School twenty minutes' drive from our neighbourhood. It was reported that Zeke kept spinning himself around in the playground. He was given a weighted jacket to wear during outdoor play times. This item was meant to 'discourage' that spinning behaviour. For fidgeting on the carpet, he was given an orthopaedic bubble cushion to sit on to 'stop' that behaviour.

During this time Zeke would pinch and pull mine and his dad's skin on our arms and bite us when we made certain requests of him, and at times, for no obvious reason. Sometimes, he would thump his dad on the head with all his strength. This behaviour stopped when he was sixteen years old after we had transitioned him to Haringey Sixth Form College.

Between the ages of four and ten years, whilst shopping with him in supermarkets, he would throw himself on the floor whilst screaming out loud. This behaviour drew attention to himself and made his father and me feel embarrassed.

From age seven to eighteen, whenever he saw any dogs, even very small poodles being carried in their owners' arms, he would scream out loudly and run away. This behaviour would at times put him in danger, since he would run into commuters, even babies being pushed along in their buggies by an adult. The worst scenario at times was when he would attempt to run out into the busy roads with oncoming traffic in sight.

He would escape from the house through the front and back doors. If these doors were locked with the key, he would attempt to climb out of closed upstairs bedroom windows.

He could not be left to play alone in the back garden because he would climb the fences and go into the neighbour's garden. On two occasions, he climbed the fence and was missing for ten minutes. While family members were out looking for him Jean, one of our next-door neighbours, who has since passed away, thought she heard a cat upstairs. When she went to investigate she found Zeke upstairs in her bedroom rampaging through her chest of drawers.

Up to age 16, Zeke did not accept 'No' as an answer from his parents. I am not sure if he did not understand the meaning of that word, did not hear the word, or if he was being defiant. Now, when he is told 'No' he usually responds, 'A change!' or 'Cancel' before he adheres to our command of 'No.'

ZEKE'S MOST PLEASANT BEHAVIOURS
Whilst I was the manager of a day-care centre for children, and he was seven to ten years old, Zeke would watch through the window to see when I had arrived home on the days that I was scheduled to work. Upon seeing me park the car, he would rush to the bathroom and start setting the bath for me. He would proceed to put out my night clothes. If I didn't go straight to the bathroom, he would insist by saying, 'Mummy, up you get, bathroom.'

As he got older, aged about 10, he would make me a cup of tea as I sat relaxing on the sofa watching the television. From his teen years he started preparing English breakfast and lunch for me at times when I was hungry and tired.

Zeke came over and kissed me on the cheeks after I had finished telling his father that he had been given a place at Haringey 6th Form College in June 2015.

MY 'AH-AH' MOMENT WITH MY SON'S AUTISM AND CONSTANT 'EARS' ISSUES

During the summer of 2017 when Zeke was 19 years and 9 months old, I made an observation which will forever change the effect of autism on the life and development of my son. A company called Isagenix produces two products which I began taking for myself. After two doses I noticed a positive change in my level of attention, focus, speech fluency, and a huge increase in my confidence level, tolerance of difficult situations in my personal life, and an improved calmness within myself.

I started to reflect on Zeke's general ability and wondered to myself if it was possible for these two products to give Zeke a better quality of life. Quite naturally I thought of his age compared to mine in determining how much of these products I should administer to my son. I began by comparing the dosages I was taking with the difference in our ages.

Each morning as a first drink I measured out the product liquid for myself, 3 tablespoons, and then mixed it with 3 tablespoons of boiled, cooled down water. I drank this drink in three gulps. I would next wait forty-five minutes before having my light breakfast.

After two weeks of continuously drinking the Isagenix mixture, I decided to introduce this same drink to Zeke. Instead of giving him the same dose as I was drinking, I mixed only one tablespoon of Isagenix. I noted after twenty-four hours that Zeke initiated a conversation. He appeared calmer and a lot more accepting of routine changes.

I decided to have a 'back to back cleanse' using Isagenix Nourish for Life cleanse. When I speak of 'back to back cleanse,' I mean that I would drink a full bottle of this Nourish over two consecutive days. Whilst doing this I would be on fasting from morning and only break my fast for the evening meal.

The only drink I would have during each fasting day is the Nourish for Life diluted with 2 litres of cold water. If I was feeling thirsty, I would quench my thirst by drinking pure water. On the second day of starting the Nourish for Life, I repeated my action of the first day. On the day after taking my 'flush out,' I was onto something significant in an excellent way. So, I began to think that this product would no doubt be of benefit to Zeke. However, I waited until he was at home for the summer holiday in 2016.

I decided to administer to Zeke 1 tablespoon of Isagenix mixed with 1 tablespoon of cooled, boiled water which was given to him daily, over a period of two weeks. During this time, his 6th Form College in Haringey was still in session before the summer holidays. I instructed Zeke to drink in two gulps, as I did when taking the Isagenix, and then he waited fifteen minutes before eating his breakfast and having his usual drink of fruit juice, mint tea or water. The first time was challenging for Zeke, but once I explained the possible benefits to him in the way where it would help him to become a better speaker, he began to have his daily dosage without any hassle.

On the Wednesday during the second week of his summer

holidays I decided that the time was right for Zeke to have his bottle of cleanse. Unlike for myself, I decided not to give Zeke a 'back to back' cleanse.

I gave him only one bottle of Nourish for Life to drink until dinner time, when I would allow him to break his fasting. At breakfast time, I mixed the 50ml of Nourish for Life into two 50ml bottles of plain water. I sat Zeke down at the dining table and explained to him the benefits of that drink. I told him that he had some rubbish in his body system that needed to be cleaned out and that this drink would clean him out. I also explained that when he finished drinking all of this drink, he would feel much better in himself.

The first sip started with a frown on the brow of his head, but it soon disappeared, and he started drinking it normally. I thought he would like it because it is quite a pleasant drink to have. I explain that he was not allowed to eat anything until dinner time and that whenever he was feeling hungry he should have some of that drink. I was surprised he did not attempt to pinch my arm like he normally does when I make a request of him. He simply said 'Ok' and went off to his room. As he walked away, I reminded him to tell me when he was ready for another of his special drink. Again, he replied, 'Ok'.

Zeke was okay drinking only his Nourish for Life flush until 12 noon, his usual lunch time. I repeated to him that he had another four hours to go before dinner time, so he should have another drink of the Nourish for Life. After he had consumed what seemed like five drinks of the Nourish for

Life, I remembered about another product called 'Snacks' that was recommended to me by my Isagenix supervisor. 'Snacks' are essentially a food supplement which also builds up the energy level in the recipient. So I fetched the bottle from my kitchen cupboard and gave three snack buttons to Zeke to eat.

Zeke ate these with delight, partly because they are round and look and taste like chocolate. These chocolate buttons seemed to have done the trick for Zeke. So, I asked him if he would like to go swimming with his support worker, Nathaniel, who had by now arrived to give me four hours respite time or relief from my caring duties with Zeke. Within minutes Zeke had packed his swimming kit, and they were both off to go swimming.

While they were gone I made sure I cooked the dinner so that upon their return dinner would be ready for Zeke to break his fast. Both Nathaniel and Zeke returned from swimming at 3.30pm that day. Dinner was ready, served and waiting on the table for them to enjoy as soon as they returned. As soon as Zeke opened the door, he could smell the aroma from the roast lamb, boiled rice, and steamed vegetables, so he reacted with 'mmmmmmmmmm', dropped his bag in the hall way, washed his hands then came and sat down at the dining table, and started serving out his dinner onto his plate. Nathaniel joined him, and they both sat and ate a hearty meal.

When they had finished eating, they both took the initiative to cover the remaining food and cleaned the table, scraped the leftovers from their plates into the bin, and stacked the used utensils to the side of the kitchen sink. Zeke said to me and Nathaniel, 'Bed sleep. Bye Nathaniel,' and went off to his bedroom. I told Nathaniel that if he wished, I would be happy for him to leave, but he should sign out at the booked time because Zeke thinks he's done enough for the day. Nathaniel said that he agreed and got up from the sofa straight away and signed himself out, then said, 'See you tomorrow, Mrs Velora.' Ten minutes after Nathaniel left, I went upstairs to check on Zeke. He was fast asleep and he did not awaken until 7:30 pm, three hours later.

For the first time in a long time, Zeke woke up and came straight downstairs, relaxed on the sofa, and watched a television programme without been prompted to do so. There was an aura of calmness about him. Not only was he calm, but he was making a real attempt to talk to me about other missing family members. He wanted to know when his father would be home, if his niece was at nursery, if his brother Cuffie was at work, and if his sister Kelsey was still pregnant. I was amazed but kept our conversation going. It was my 'Eureka' moment!!! My son has shown tremendous improvement in his communication skills, and I knew the Isagenix products I had been giving to him were to be credited for this progress.

As a result, I have decided that three times each year, I will administer these products to him: during the Christmas holidays, Easter and summer. During the summer I will be giving him a Nourish for Life cleanse for two days, but during the other two holidays he will only be given one cleanse.

Since these initiatives, Zeke's father and I have observed tremendous progress in Zeke's speech and behaviour. He is making a real effort to speak with us and adhering to routine. His concentration and understanding of things in general are also improved.

After a two-week lapse since Zeke was given the Isagenix products, he had started to plug his ears with screwed up tissues and kept telling us that his ears were aching. I looked over at his father and said, 'When are these doctor's appointments, repeated prescription and syringe going to stop?' I mourned. 'This has been going on since he was four years old. We really need to seek out alternative herbal medicine for this eczema he keeps getting in his ears. Syringing his ears so often, six times per year, can't be good for his ear drum,', I complained.

I went into a deep conversation about the aloe vera plant gel I was given to use by a Rastafarian fisherman back in Jamaica a few years ago. It was to be used to treat the terrible skin rash he had developed whilst we were on holiday in Jamaica when he was seven years old. I had experienced another 'Eureka' moment. I quickly got up from the sofa and said to my husband, 'You know what? I'm going over to Wood Green shopping centre to see what I can find for Zeke's eczema ears problem.' The journey from my home took me thirty minutes. I could think of nothing else but how well and quickly this pulp from the aloe vera plant had cured the rash all over Zeke's body. As I parked my car in Morrison's car park in Wood Green, I had a thought to go into Holland and Barrett's to make some enquiries about the natural form of the aloe vera gel.

'Eureka!' After speaking to three different staff members, a young, fair-haired, pale-skinned male member of staff showed me to the closest they had to the aloe vera gel I was looking for. He explained to me that because the skin surface in the ear is different to that of our outer body he couldn't say it would be as effective if used in the ear as when used on the outer skin of our bodies. As usual, he instructed me to take him to be examined by the GP who should be able to prescribe the best product for his ears. But I had already had enough of the GP's prescriptions. Whatever products were given by the GP were only very temporary, about every six weeks. So, I said to the young man, 'This is just the product I've been looking for.' I paid for it and left the shop with the hope and belief that this product would cure the eczema in my son's ears. I took it home, showed it to his father and explained to him how I planned to use it in Zeke's ears.

I called Zeke from upstairs and I told him to come and sit beside me on the sofa. I asked him if his ears were still hurting him, and he replied, 'Yes, ears hurting,' whilst cupping his left hand over his left ear. I showed him the aloe vera product that I had bought. I also showed him the cotton buds that I had bought. I removed the cover from the tube of the aloe vera gel and explained to him, 'I am squirting out a little bit of this gel into the cover of the tube and will scoop some of the gel into the lid. Then, I will use the cotton bud to scoop up the gel and use the cotton bud to swish it around in your ears.' He watched and listened well. He remained quite still for me to apply the gel into both his ears. When I had finished applying the gel in both ears, he picked up a clean cotton bud and pushed it into both ears, twirling it around into his ears as if I had missed certain parts in his ears that needed to be reached.

For reassurance that I'm doing the right thing I will limit myself to applying this aloe gel to Zeke's inner ear only when he complains of having an ear ache. On these occasions I will do it only for three days, twice daily. Every three months I will have the GP check Zeke's inner ears for infection and eczema. On the first occasion that I had the GP examine Zeke's ears she looked surprised then she remarked 'this is the best condition I've seen his ears in'. 'The eczema has cleared up'. I proceeded to explain to her about the product I've started using in Zeke's ears. The GP took a deep breath then said I think you should continue to use that product in his ears whenever he complains about having ear ache. 'I'm always willing to continue checking his ears whenever you feel its necessary.

CHAPTER 10:
From birth to 21 months

"IT is never too late to expand the mind of a person on the autism spectrum" Temple Grandin

Zeke was a gorgeous baby boy, so much so that our immediate family all started calling him 'Gorgeous' and continued doing so well up until he was five months old. He even started responding to that name more readily than when he was called by his real name, Zeke. I was happy that he was achieving his developmental milestones. At two weeks he was following my movements with his eyes. By four weeks he was able to follow me by moving his head from left to right. By six weeks he was able to hold my finger and pull himself up towards me.

By three months he was able to remain in a sitting upright position when propped up with two pillows. By five months he was sitting up unsupported. By six months he was pulling himself up onto his hands and knees and starting to crawl around. At seven months he was crawling and was able to pull himself up from a sitting position to a standing position by holding onto an object for support.

By eleven months he was walking and using single words

such as 'mummy', 'daddy', 'babba', 'sister', 'Trevor', 'cat', 'dog'. He was also able to repeat single words when requested. By 14 months he was able to string two words together to make a sentence such as 'my ball', 'my shoes', 'my car', 'daddy shoes', and 'Mummy shoes'. By 18 months he was able to read environmental prints such as Mc Donald's, Burger King, Tesco etc. And, at 21 months, he was able to name the characters in a story book. He was able to sing a few nursery rhymes such as *Baa baa black sheep, have you any wool?*

FROM 21 MONTHS TO FIVE YEARS
Shortly after my son's second birthday, we were visited at our home by a health professional to carry out routine observation and assessment on him. Her questions were mainly based around how he played. She made notes as I describe to her the way in which he lined up his building blocks horizontally as opposed to vertically in the way our first and second born did when they were at his age. She wanted to know how many words he had in his vocabulary and if he had started stringing words together to form short sentences. She seemed annoyed when he walked into her as opposed to walking around her when he wanted to get to the other side of her.

It became obvious to me towards the middle of her visit that she had concerns about our son's development. But she was not making any attempt to divulge any information to me or the intensity of her concerns. She suggested that she would be speaking with our GP with the intention of arranging an appointment for him to be assessed by a paediatrician at the hospital.

Up to this point I was oblivious about the fact that our son was showing symptoms of autism. No professional involved with the care of our son informed us that our son had autistic tendencies.

Within three weeks, an appointment was sent from the hospital for our son. During this initial appointment with the paediatrician, different parts of his body were measured and a series of blood tests were done.

Beryl, from the 'home tuition centre' in Enfield, was appointed to visit our home in order to do one-to-one work with him over a period of eight weeks.

I decided to monitor closely how well he was using words. I asked the rest of the family to do the same and we communicated these words to each other. We also began to make a real effort to encourage him to repeat after us more words than usual. His father, sister, brother and I became a proper team working together to encourage Zeke's speech development. We started to reflect on what could have possibly caused Zeke to develop autism. At this time, meningitis was affecting very young children nationwide. As a family we all started to read up on the symptoms of meningitis and also on autism and to share our newly found knowledge with each other.

At eight months our son started to attend a local kindergarten, but within six weeks of attendance, he became seriously ill with a high temperature, red spots all over his body and he had convulsions. He was kept away from the nursery for six weeks until he had recovered and was able to return to the nursery. We began to focus on the skin rash, high fever, runny nose and bodily shakes or convulsions he developed after attending kindergarten in Edmonton for only six weeks. He became so obviously ill one night that the whole family drove him off to hospital.

When he returned to the nursery, I asked for an appointment to speak to the manager in order to share with her my concerns that our son may have picked up a virus from the nursery. I was surprised at the response that the manager gave to me.

She angrily said to me that it looks like I'm trying to create trouble for her staff, and as a result she told me that I should take my child and leave the premises. I tried to explain to her that causing trouble was not my intention. I was simply trying to make her aware of my concerns that other children may also have picked up the virus. But she was insistent that I withdraw my child from the nursery and place him elsewhere. I then decided to ask my sister Nevaeh, living in Islington, to take care of our son. After two weeks she said to me that she would no longer be able to care for him and that I should find a childminder closer to my home. I telephoned the childminder networks office and asked them for a list of childminders in my local borough.

My husband and I decided upon a Turkish lady. After three months this lady told me one afternoon, after I'd had a hectic day in the classroom, that she could no longer take care of Zeke. Zeke was now 17 months old and had started to call her 'mummy' and her husband 'daddy'. I had no further choice but to attempt to look for another childminder as I had committed myself to a one-year contract in a lovely small primary school.

Luckily I had kept the original list of names of childminders given to me six months previously. I read through the list again and decided to ring the lady whose track record and facility looked the most desirable. To my disappointment she said that she didn't have a vacancy but that she knew of another childminder who had a vacancy. So, she recommended a lady with a surname starting with T. I continued to search in the meantime. I started looking down the list of childminders and I came across the name of an English-sounding lady by the name Mrs S, and I liked her track record.

I then decided to telephone Mrs S before telephoning Ms T, but I wasn't satisfied with her softly spoken, conservative voice. So I proceeded to telephone Ms T, whose voice was strong and confident. When she told me that she actually had one vacancy, I was elated and decided that I should give her a visit first. When I arrived at Ms T's home, I was happy to see that she had other toddlers in her care who were only a few months older than Zeke - a boy and a girl who took an instant liking to Zeke and started playing with him. I was dissatisfied that her three dogs stayed in the house with the children. But the other two children did not mind and neither did Zeke.

As Ms T and I chatted all three toddlers took turns stroking the dogs which seemed to have been enjoying the affection and attention they were being given. Although I had given Ms T my word that she was the one I had chosen to take care of my son, I also told her that out of courtesy I would be going to visit another childminder I had booked an appointment with before I called her. Ms T agreed that was the decent thing to do.

On the day I visited this other lady I did not bring Zeke along with me to meet her, purely because I had decided that Ms T was going to be his childminder. After explaining to the lady that I had already chosen someone else she asked who that person was. When I said 'Ms T' she remarked that she knew her and added that Ms T had recently spent some time in hospital due to a serious illness. Having heard her comment I became a little bit concerned about Ms T and felt that she might not be well enough to give Zeke the level of care and stimulation he needed for a normal active toddler.

On reflection on how calm and interactive Ms T was on the day of my visit with all three toddlers, I felt that perhaps this other childminder was being vindictive and only wanted me to change my mind and allow her to become Zeke's childminder. I thanked her and explained to her that had I visited her first I probably would not have bothered to visit Ms T. So, Ms T was now entrusted with the care and stimulation of my precious toddler whilst I returned to my teaching position three days per week.

I was never totally happy with the idea of any of my children being cared for by someone I hardly knew. Fortunately, Kelsey and Cuffie were cared for by my sister Nevaeh and one of

AUTISM – ONE FAMILY'S JOURNEY

her friends when they were small. But that's the situation with which I was faced and unfortunately had no control over it. My husband's income alone could not sustain all the requirements to run a happy home and provide for three children. Zeke seemed very happy going to his childminder that year from April to July 2000, when the school holidays began. He had become very popular with child E and J, the other two toddlers also being cared for by Ms T.

I was extremely happy when the summer holidays arrived because I knew I would have six weeks with my three precious children. Ms T by now was saying that Zeke was calling her by her real name and that her ten-year-old son Jack he was calling daddy. She remarked that her sixteen-year-old daughter Georgette was crazy about him and kept saying how cute he was. I was happy for the positive feedback that I was receiving from Ms T as I said, 'Bye for now' to her while Zeke also smiled at her and said, 'Bye-bye'.

Two weeks later Zeke received the MMR vaccination suggested by our GP, Dr L, since Zeke would be visiting France, a country which we had visited once before when Zeke was 10 months old. I was quite reluctant for him to have the triple MMR jab, but I trusted the advice of my GP, since she was an excellent doctor. One week after receiving the MMR, our family of five travelled by the Eurostar to spend one week at Disneyland in Paris.

Two days into our holiday, on the third morning, I noticed that Zeke was not his usual chirpy, chatty and cuddly self. I gave him a bath and dressed him as usual before leaving our hotel apartment to take the five-minute walk to the communal dining room for breakfast. As Zeke seemed so sad and clingy, his father Zephie decided to carry him in his arms. Zeke rested his head on his dad's shoulder and did not utter a sound or called anyone's name as he had been doing since he was nine months old. I knew that there was something wrong but did not think it was serious. By now it was ten days since he had been given the MMR injections.

I thought that perhaps his thigh, where he had received the injection, was aching and sore. I looked in the distance for a suitable location for us to be seated. I spotted one, and I suggested to my husband that he take the children to that particular table while I went and collected a high chair into which Zeke could sit. When I returned to the dining table with the high chair, I carefully removed Zeke from his father's arms and gently placed him in the high chair. Because of his overall clinginess, I very carefully strapped him in it. When Zephie, Kelsey and Cuffie had decided to join the queue for the buffet breakfast, I asked them to bring some for Zeke and me. They gladly agreed.

The queue moved at a steady and quick pace, and within fifteen minutes Zephie and the other two children had returned to our breakfast table with both a cooked English breakfast and cereal for all of us to eat to our contentment. We all knew that Zeke liked Ready brek cereal, so I poured some hot milk on his cereal, gently mixed it in, scooped up a small amount onto the spoon and brought it towards his mouth. He opened his mouth and received the serving of cereal before swallowing. I gently removed the spoon from his mouth, and he started chewing on the cereal before swallowing. He was clearly hungry so I did not hesitate to place a second serving into his half-opened mouth whilst he appeared to be looking in the distance at two other toddlers sitting and chatting away to their parents. Again, I removed the spoon from his mouth, leaving him to chew his cereal before swallowing.

By now the cup of tea which my husband Zephie had poured and mixed for me was getting cold, so I handed the spoon to Zeke and said to him, 'Come on Zeke, you can feed yourself. Take the spoon.' Zeke, who the family had agreed was obviously right-handed, did not even attempt to lift his right hand to take the spoon from me. Instead he just looked at me and then looked at the rest of his family. We were all showing concern for him by saying words such as 'Zeke, what's wrong?' 'Come on, eat your cereal.' 'It's nice,' 'Mmmm.'

I managed to have two sips of my tea before I decided to gently physically lift up Zeke's right hand to place the spoon in his hand. As I lifted up his hand, he made a high-pitched scream as if he was experiencing severe pain from that hand. He lifted the left hand as if to bar me from touching his right hand.

We all became concerned that perhaps the joint of his right arm was dislocated. We were all concerned that something was seriously wrong with Zeke and that he urgently needed medical attention. I suggested that we should all return to our hotel apartment and from there use the phone to request a visit from the resort nurse. Within ten minutes a team of paramedics were knocking on the front door of our apartment, two females and one male. All spoke very good English but they also spoke French, which only Kelsey had an idea what they were saying to each other.

After taking a brief personal and medical history of Zeke, including a question, 'Is he up to date with all his immunisations?' the male member of the team suggested that he would like to escort us all over to the local hospital. He explained that at the local hospital Zeke could have a thorough checkup and maybe an x-ray of his right shoulder. Within fifteen minutes of arriving at the hospital, the female nurse remaining with us escorted us into a consulting room where we were met by two male doctors who introduced themselves to us, one as the Registrar and the other as a paediatrician. My husband and I made piercing eye contact with each other because we both sensed an air of efficiency and a genuine concern for what could possibly be wrong with Zeke.

Reflex actions tests were carried out on Zeke before he was escorted next door to the radiography room to have an x-ray done of his shoulder. The result showed that his shoulder was not broken. But it did show some dislocation of the tendon in his elbow joint. The paediatrician gently held out Zeke's right hand and used his own thumb to apply pressure in the middle of the elbow joint of Zeke's right arm. Then he used his other hand to gently move Zeke's right hand up and down in two movements only. Afterwards he said, 'Problem is solved. You can all return to your hotel and enjoy the remainder of your holiday.' With all that said and done Zeke lifted up both hands to his dad and said, 'Daddy up'. So his dad picked him up and we all walked back with the two paramedics to the ambulance, who escorted us all back to the Euro Disney complex.

Although Zeke was now able to lift both hands and used his right hand to feed himself, since then he has never been the chirpy, chatty, and cooperative toddler he was on arrival in France.

In September 2000 after returning from France, Zeke returned to his child minder Ms T. Ms T. began to regularly report to me when I arrived to pick him up after work that Zeke was constantly trying to climb through her car window while she was driving. She informed me that he did not listen to her and that he was not doing as he was told as before. She also informed me that he was laughing at her and making her feel incapable or inferior.

At home we also observed Zeke's current behaviour, so we had to decide what we could do to help to break these habits. The Light and Sound Centre was highly recommended, so we arranged an appointment for these professionals to assist us with Zeke's behaviour. After discussing my concerns with the centre manager that Zeke was not hearing clearly, I was advised to play classical music softly at nights in Zeke's bedroom. I was told that the vibrations from the music would stimulate his ear drum and improve hearing and listening as well as make him less irritable.

I now began to have vivid dreams such as the following: One night I dreamt that I took Zeke to be assessed by a specialist developmental psychologist. In this dream he described to me that Zeke would not be able to learn to write, and he drew a pattern to explain to me why he knows why Zeke would not be able to learn to write. However, this has not been the case as Zeke has learnt to write even though it is 'infant script style', and he is now 20 years old.

From 18 months old to five years old, I kept regular records of words and expressions that Zeke had used. I did this as a means to monitor how much progress he was making in his speech development. This process of recording was good for my sanity and gave me hope. Samples of these recordings can be found in Chapter 11.

At age three Zeke went under a general anaesthetic for circumcision, which is a process whereby the foreskin of his penis got removed. He was found to have a condition called 'balanitis'. The medics felt that the operation was necessary because the foreskin of his penis was hanging too far down. They felt he would become more prone to getting infections in the penis area because this condition would make it difficult for him to wash and keep that area of his penis clean.

DENTAL CARE
Due to Zeke's hyperactive behaviour, he had missed out on vital dental care because he would not settle on a dentist's

chair to allow them to examine his teeth, nor allow them to carry out minor treatment. When he was two years old, I became concerned about his premolars because his breath had become unpleasant. I knew the front teeth and incisors were fine because I could see those easily. I was convinced that the back teeth were causing problems. I booked an appointment for our family dentist in Finsbury Park to examine his teeth. The task of getting him to sit on the dentist's chair was very trying, but we managed. We managed to coax him to sit on the dentist's chair. The minute that the dentist said, 'Zeke, open your mouth and let's see what's wrong,' It was embarrassing to hear how loud he was screaming. He plainly refused to allow the dentist to look into his mouth.

The dentist was patient with him and persevered for about fifteen minutes, trying his best to coerce Zeke to open his mouth wide for him to examine his teeth. In the end the dentist gave up and asked, 'Is he one of those kids?' I knew exactly what he meant, so I said, 'He's still undergoing medical investigations, but it looks like the observations and feedback is leading to a diagnosis of autism.'

After all this drama the dentist said, 'He needs to have an appointment with the Primary Care Trust in the borough where you are living.' I said, 'How should I go about doing that?' My dentist replied, 'You don't need to do anything straight away. I'm going to write a letter to them so all you need to do is to wait to hear from them.' He went on to say that he would be very surprised if I didn't get an appointment within two weeks. He advised me to try my best to assist Zeke when brushing his teeth. He also wrote a prescription for mouthwash which he wanted Zeke to use in the mornings before breakfast and in the evenings before going to bed.

As the dentist had predicted, I was sent an appointment for Zeke to be examined by a dentist at the Primary Care Trust. They wanted him to attend their dental practice within two days of the date on the letter. Zeke was now three years old, and the bad breath was still noticeable, so I was glad to receive the early appointment. I tried my best to explain to Zeke about his visit to this other dentist. He repeated the word 'dentist' after me and he did not seem distressed about his appointment. However, during his visit to the dentist, again he would not cooperate with the dentist's requests. After several attempts by the dentist to get Zeke to open his mouth for him to examine his teeth, which Zeke vigorously resisted, after thirty minutes the dentist gave up and said he would give him another appointment in six weeks' time.

I took him for his appointment six weeks later, and he still would not allow the dentist to examine his mouth, so he sent him away again. This time, the dentist gave Zeke another appointment for him to attend in three months' time. A week before Zeke was due to attend this appointment, I received a cancellation letter. This letter stated that the dentist had left the practice and that they were waiting to appoint a new dentist. Six months later we received another appointment, which I was surprised to get. When we arrived at the dental practice, I was told that Zeke would be seen by the dental hygienist. The dental hygienist was a hugely pregnant lady, and she was calm and more patient with Zeke. She explained and demonstrated the best way to brush his teeth, to which he was very cooperative as he looked at his teeth in the mirror.

The dentist explained that Zeke did have some cavities in two upper premolars as well as in two lower premolars, but that she was not going to recommend any treatment straight away. She said she would like to examine his teeth again in six months' time. However, she advised me to continue to assist Zeke when brushing his teeth. Twelve months had gone by and Zeke had not been sent another follow-up appointment, so I telephoned the Primary Care Trust and made enquiries as to why Zeke had not been sent a dental appointment. I explained that it was twelve months since he had last seen the dentist.

The receptionist apologised and commented that they had been having difficulties recruiting a new dentist for that particular dental practice in Edmonton Green. She reassured me that she would do her best to get an appointment sent out to Zeke as soon as possible. Within four weeks, I received a phone call from Evergreen Dental Practice in Edmonton Green. The receptionist had a Caribbean accent and was quite pleasant to speak with. She explained that an appointment was actually sent out for Zeke six weeks earlier, but Zeke did not attend. When I explained to her that it was not sent to our address, she seemed baffled and said that two appointments were sent but neither appointment was attended by Zeke.

I concluded by saying, 'I don't know which address those appointment letters were sent to, but they definitely did not come to our address.' She then said, 'Let's try and make another appointment for him.' The first appointment was treated as urgent, so he was given one for the following week. By now, Zeke was five years old. This time round, Zeke was quite cooperative with the dentist. He actually allowed her to put a probe into his mouth to examine his teeth with very little fuss.

It took her thirty minutes to complete a thorough examination of Zeke's mouth and teeth. When she had finished she told me that Zeke had four badly decayed teeth and that she was not even going to attempt filling them. She recommended that they should be removed as soon as possible because they must be causing him a lot of pain. At the end of that sentence, she then said that the best way to remove them was under general anaesthetic at the local hospital. She told me that I would receive an appointment from the hospital soon, because she was treating it as urgent. Two weeks later I received an appointment for Zeke to attend the hospital Day Ward to have the extractions done.

He was to be 'nil by mouth' for at least two hours before his procedure. The day finally came for Zeke to undergo surgery for tooth extraction. I tried my best to explain to Zeke about the procedure. He repeated 'dentist' and 'hospital' after me, and seemed calm about it. At the hospital he was well behaved and cooperated with the doctors after he had received the anaesthetic. Both the dentist and the anaesthetist were very gentle and kind with him. The entire procedure took forty-five minutes, and when he had awakened, within five minutes he was returned to me in the recovery suite. We were then told to remain in the recovery suite for one hour before leaving. Zeke said he wanted a drink, so I gave him firstly a sip of water then a box of orange juice.

Within forty-five minutes of being in recovery Zeke was clearly awake and ready to leave, but I wanted to honour the medic's advice. I directed Zeke to the small play house in the corner of the room. Zeke was happy to play there until I said, 'Let's go, Zeke; it's time to go,' so he stopped playing and held my hand. We walked together to the carpark and got home fifteen minutes later. It was a relief for me to know that Zeke was no longer having tooth ache.

The bad breath was noticeably reduced, but first thing in the morning his breath was still noticeably unpleasant, although not as much as before the extraction of his decayed teeth. I concluded that there must be a problem with his tonsils and sinus because the unpleasant smell was also coming from his nostrils. I concluded that Zeke had lived with tooth ache for nearly two years. My only comfort was that this experience would make him into a resilient young man, although I strongly believed that no child should have suffered a toothache for such a lengthy period of time.

Whilst attending the local primary school nursery, I was approached by a mother who had observed Zeke's behaviour. She suggested that Zeke would benefit from being seen by a therapist at the Osteopathic Centre. The Osteopathic Centre was in Old Street and was highly recommended to me by this mother. From the age of four to seven, Zeke was receiving therapy from these professionals. After receiving the contact detail from this mother, I did not hesitate to contact the Centre and set up an appointment. Our first appointment involved giving the therapist Zeke's medical and family history.

I was surprised at Zeke's final assessment results. I was reassured by the Osteopathic secretary that Zeke could be helped by the therapists there. Firstly the therapist explained to me that the fontanelle of Zeke's skull had closed up too early after he was born. This action is known as Scaphocephaly. As a result the skull was squashing his brain and was causing a lot of problems with his learning and behaviour.

I was also informed that he had a severe hearing infection, and that it could be treated by 'touch therapy'. It was described to me that within Zeke's body system there was baby excretion that was trapped in his body and that by using 'touch therapy' on specific areas of his back, this toxicity could be released. The therapist went on to explain that the toxicity would have the appearance of a 'yellow stool or faeces' similar to the type that young babies pass out before they are introduced to puréed food from about the age of four months old.

Surprisingly to me, within a week, when Zeke was about five years old he did excrete that yellow-looking stool.

In regards to the severe ear infection, at age six years an MRI scan of Zeke's head did reveal that he had a severe inner ear and nose infection. However the hospital staff didn't report the true result of this scan to our GP or to me. Instead he was discharged from the clinic with a report that stated 'no abnormalities' was found. Due to my determination, one year later I requested a second opinion on that same scan imaging. On this occasion it was reported that the MRI scan showed that Zeke had a paranasal disease which included a diseased sinus. Zeke also had nodules on his voice box and enlarged tonsils. As a result two weeks later, Zeke underwent a three-in-one operation to have his inner ear, adenoids cleaned out and grommets inserted in the Eustachian tubes as they were too narrow. His adenoids and tonsils were also removed.

CHAPTER 11:
The continuation of my autism journey

"If you want to be the best, you have to do things that other people aren't willing to do." Michael Phelps.

Here are some excerpts from my home observations and reports of Zeke from April 2001 to September 2004.
1. Monday 9 April 2001 - Zeke called his name tonight while going to pick up a marble in the corner of his bedroom.
2. Saturday 14 April 2001 - Today Zeke said, 'This is a ball.' 'My ball.' 'Some.' 'Here.' 'Share.'
3. Tuesday 17 April 2001 - Zeke said 'Why?' He also bent down at the door, looked at the bolt and said, 'This is…?' He also kept waving at his shadow and said to himself, 'Hello, hello, and hello.'
4. Wednesday 18 April - Zeke said, 'Paper.'
5. Thursday 19 April - Zephie said that Zeke looked at himself in the mirror and kept saying, 'Hello! Hello!'
6. Monday 23 April 2001 - Trevor reported that Zeke said, 'Thank you' to him when he was given his dinner. Zeke also said, 'up' to me when I resisted getting up to go to the kitchen with him.

7. Monday 30 April 2001 - Florence reported that Zeke behaved well. He also sat with her and looked at her as she pointed out the names of the different pictures to him. Whenever she said, 'Zeke, come here,' he went to her. When she asked him to give something to her he went straight away and gave it to her. Zeke tapped Cuffie on the knee and said, 'Hya.'
8. Tuesday 1 May 2001- I told Zeke to 'Stay there,' meaning, 'Stay in the bath.' When I left the bathroom, Zeke repeated 'Stay there,' quietly.
9. Sunday 5 May 2001 - Zeke gave me the bottle and said 'Ta!' I also told Zeke to shut the door and he shut it straightaway.
10. Sunday 6 May 2001 - Zeke touched the football design on Cuffie's pyjama and said, 'Mine!' This was heard by Cuffie and Trevor.
11. Tuesday 8 May 2001 - Zeke saw a young black lady walking along the road and he shouted to her, 'Trishie!' Zeke also looked at the cow in the puzzle and said, 'How you doing?'
12. Wednesday 9 May 2001 - Zeke went to put the key in Nevaeh's front door and said, 'A door!' He also picked up Ossie's phone, pressed the button then put the phone to his ear and said, 'Hullo!' Zephie said that as soon as Zeke arrived at Nevaeh's front door he kept saying, 'Hullo! Hullo! Hullo!'
13. Thursday 10 May 2001 - Zeke said 'Run!' when he saw the horse race on television.

14. Staff D from Leapfrog reported that Zeke's eye contact was improving today and that he sat well for circle time.
15. Wednesday 16 May 2001 - Nevaeh reported that Zeke kept repeating, 'Trishie, Trishie, and Trishie' a lot today.
16. Thursday 17 May 2001 - Staff S and D at Leapfrog nursery reported that Zeke enjoyed the parachute today. He even went and pulled another boy's hand and directed him to the parachute. Unfortunately the boy refused to go. They also pointed out that Zeke has a good pencil hold. He also engaged in a variety of activities. His eye contact is also getting better. He gives fleeting eye contact when he wants something.
17. Friday 18 May 2001 - Staff B at playgroup explained to me that Zeke wanted a doll that was too high for him to reach. So he got her by the hand and took her to get it down for him. She concluded that if he knows to do this, then the words will soon be added. Staff B also said that Zeke said something which sounded like, 'Thank you.' She also said that Zeke joined in with songs and movements, which he enjoyed immensely. Manager L the added that Zeke is now enjoying nursery.
18. Sunday 20 May 2001 - Zeke stretched for the salad bowl and said, 'A mine.'
19. Tuesday 22 May 2001 - At 7.30am Zeke went into Cuffie's room and stayed about 10 minutes until I called him. He came out immediately and said, 'Cuffie, Dad, my mamam.' Later on today at Leapfrog nursery the speech therapist

told Cuffie that Zeke is maintaining a lot more eye contact and is interacting more with other children. The staff also described how Zeke enjoyed playing football outside and even attempted to fetch the ball when it had gone over the fence.

20. Wednesday 23 May 2001 - Kelsey reported that when she flashed a biscuit in front of Zeke he said, 'Biscuit, biscuit, ta!'
21. Tuesday 29 May 2001 - Whilst watching Teletubbies, Zeke copied them when they said 'Boo!' (as in 'peek a boo!').
22. Friday 1 June 2001 - at 2am Zeke sat on the potty chanting, 'Poo, Poo, and Poo'.
23. Sunday 3 June 2001 - When someone tried to take something from Zeke he resisted and said, 'No' and 'Oh God.'
24. Sunday 10 June 2001 - Took Zeke to Tumble Tots in Edgware (first session). He enjoyed this very much but did not seem to listen much to the guide's instructions or keep to the suggested apparatus in the circuit. Next time I will insist that he follow instructions and stay in the group.
25. Monday 18 June 2001 - Zeke looked me in the eyes and initiated conversation in his own language. Then paused as if waiting for my reply.
26. Tuesday 19 June 2001- Zeke woke up this a.m. saying, 'Oh no.' The speech therapist told Zephie that Zeke has improved a lot since the last time she saw him. Eye contact is very good and he interacts well with the other children.
27. Friday 29 June 2001 - Zeke in his haste to press the bell said, in what seems to be stuttering, 'Let me open the

door.' He also said, 'Woof' on seeing the dog in the advert. He played 'Peek a boo' and said 'Boo!'

28. Friday 25 January 2002 - Zeke went to nursery after 4 days off. The Ed. Psyche, said Zeke now plays a lot with the other children. She explains that he frequently goes up to them, looks into their eyes and touches their hand before taking things from them. The Ed. Psyche explained that once this kind of interaction is taking place speech will soon develop. Today she said Zeke said, 'Goal' and 'Bye-bye.'

29. Monday 28 January 2002 - I spoke with Manager L quite briefly this morning. We talked about the possibility of Zeke moving up to their mainstream nursery. Manager L said that Zeke will be attending Thursday afternoon at their mainstream nursery after half-term. Manager L also mentioned how well Zeke has come on over the last few weeks. She talked about his good eye-contact and that he now sits for story and circle time, interacts well with both staff and children, plays with other children and has started to use words in the right context. She did, however, mention that Zeke is a very emotional child. For example, he will be doing something quite happily and for no reason burst out crying as if he remembers something. The upsetting thing for them is that he won't speak so he can't tell them why he is crying.

30. Friday 8 February 2002 - I spoke briefly with Manager L and staff S this morning. They told me that they have some concerns about Zeke since the last two weeks. They said

that Zeke has been regressing slightly to some of his old behaviours. For example, he tends to want to run around a lot more than previously, he doesn't want to sit for story and snack time. He is avoiding making eye contact. He is becoming obsessive, holding onto things and won't let go of them. He is hiding things so that he can go back to them later. He keeps trying to go behind the cooker and has pushed it over once. Staff S says she is constantly saying 'No' to him and he seems to be avoiding making eye contact with her especially. Manager L wanted to know if there has been any changes at home over the last two weeks or if he has eaten any foods different from what he normally eats. Manager L stressed that they know that Zeke is a very emotional child and previously when they've sung their goodbye song in which they mentioned that Carer F is coming to pick him up he started to cry. However, they did confirm that Zeke is using a lot more words, uses the toilet independently and follows instructions more.

CHAPTER 12:
From diagnosis at age 5 to age 19.

"Building up a weakness just makes you less disabled. Building a strength can take you to the top of the world"
John Elder Robinson

The London borough in which we live has a reputation of children being diagnosed as autistic

I frequently ask myself if there is something in the atmosphere, or are most homes in my home borough haunted by a ghost, why it is that a larger amount of children are getting diagnosed as autistic in comparison to other London boroughs?

Over the last 20 years there have been many children who have been diagnosed as autistic. The findings are worrying. Even though there are many girls who are being diagnosed as autistic, this diagnosis is much higher amongst boys. But what is even more worrying is the fact that more African and Caribbean boys are being diagnosed with this condition than any other races. My findings are derived from my observation and interpretations I had made in a few of the primary schools where I've worked as a teacher and as a learning support worker.

I also acquired personal experience from my son Zeke's early years education in a local, privately managed playgroup and from his Reception and Year 1 class at a school in my home borough.

My observations confirmed to me that carers don't spend enough time interacting with certain children as they play. They don't get down to their levels when speaking with them. Instead, the staff were usually seen to be carrying out observations and writing reports on targeted children. I believe that this approach could be possible reasons as to why more children are being diagnosed as being autistic. In addition the lack of continuous support for these children was also a contributing factor. These reports were usually used as evidence so that these targeted children would be regarded as requiring speech and language therapy and consequently secure funding from the Education Authority.

SENSORY STIMULATION

After Zeke's initial two weeks' observation period at the playgroup we were invited to a review meeting for feedback. The manager reassured us that Zeke was in the right place and that they can meet his educational needs. Then she proceeded to tell us that Zeke has 'Sensory Stimulation obsession' and proceeded to explain that he has the need to stroke the skin of staff arms. I then became concerned and enquired about the seriousness of those habits and if they were treatable. She explained that there were specific activities that they will put in place to help Zeke overcome his specific sensory difficulties. These activities would include play with playdough and playing in cornflour mixture using both hands and feet. Sand and water play were also included.

After a further two weeks we were invited for another review meeting. This time we were told that Zeke was improving due to the sensory stimulation activities and that he was getting involved in all play activities. We were then informed now that during these play times, with the mixture of cornflour, that he felt the need to remove all of his clothes and cover himself all over with the mixture. The staff confirmed that he clearly needs sensory stimulation in order to assist his normal development process.

Having noted the lack of progress in Zeke's speech development at the playgroup, an incident took place at the nursery where he went missing without anyone being aware until the end of outdoor play. There was an incident where another boy had hit Zeke then Zeke hit him back. I was surprised when the manager informed me that Zeke had hit at all. I was then given the true report by one of the childcare staff, where she stated that the other boy had kept hitting Zeke and he seemed to have had enough of getting hit so he retaliated, with the attitude that the boy would not hit him again.

Before leaving Leapfrog at age three years and five months, I must confirm that Zeke by this time had regained giving good eye contact, though there was no improvement with his speech development.

AUTISM – ONE FAMILY'S JOURNEY

Zeke was officially diagnosed as having autism at the age of five in the summer term before he entered Reception class of his first primary school. Being diagnosed as autistic needed twenty-five hours of learning support with an assistant. Coming with this diagnosis the local government had put in place different streams of funding for children who have hearing disabilities. The disability allowance given to one parent to support the child or children was to be paid into a bank account every four weeks. The direct payment was to be paid into a separate bank account and to be used to employ a support worker to care for the child so that the parents could have a break. I was surprised at the information as none of the health or teaching professionals involved in Zeke's Care Plan and diagnosis had ever mentioned this to me.

What I also found to be unfair was that Zeke, who desperately needed speech therapy, did not always receive it in that the therapist would be assigned to teaching English to non-English speaking children. In addition, the support worker who would be brought in specially to support Zeke was frequently withdrawn from working with him and used as an interpreter to Turkish families and their children. At these times Zeke would be left unsupported for long periods of time. As a result he lapsed further and further behind in his English language development and his frustrations were beginning to build up. It was clear that he had not been given clear directions.

ZEKE'S PRIMARY REPORTS
KNOWLEDGE AND UNDERSTANDING OF THE WORLD

Zeke has good computer skills and uses the mouse proficiently. However, he concentrates for a few minutes on the given programme and if not watched carefully will click in and out of programmes on the desktop, showing little understanding of what he sees. Zeke is beginning to show more interest in his schedule and the class timetable. He is beginning to realise that on each day there is an order of events, e.g. 'start and finish', 'how much work' and 'when, what, next'. Zeke is aware of the difference between home and school and between different areas of the school, e.g. playground and classroom. He uses tools with adult supervision (normally the hand over hand approach) e.g. a rolling pin with dough: Zeke will put playdough in his mouth or smell and lick it. He presses his finger into the middle and rolls it in his hands. He will explore other textures such as sand, rice and pasta and enjoys water play. He loves bubbles and explores them fully, e.g. tracking, popping, and swiping. Zeke will hold the blower close to his mouth and try to blow bubbles.

CREATIVE DEVELOPMENT

Zeke must be watched at all times when using scissors as he will try to cut his lips, fingers and hair. If kept on task by an adult he will try to cut simple shapes. Zeke loves art activities and with support he can spread glue and stick art materials onto paper. He uses a paint brush well, with reminders of how he holds it or with adult support (hand-over-hand) to make a picture. He is improving his colouring skills. Zeke likes playing a variety of musical instruments and has demonstrated a good singing voice during intensive interaction sessions. He moves in time to music and loves dancing. He has favourite songs which he will sing e.g. *Who let the dogs out?* or various advertising jingles.

PHYSICAL DEVELOPMENT
Zeke is well coordinated and enjoys physical activities. He runs, jumps, climbs, rolls and descends stairs properly. He experiences some proprioceptor difficulties, which means difficulties walking in a straight line, standing on one leg etc, and will flop onto his peers or adults next to him. Zeke does not respond to adult instructions during PE lessons and has to be physically prompted to focus on what the adult is requesting e.g. 'Stop'. He has good dressing and undressing skills and can undo and do up zips, put on his coat, put on his jumper, socks and trousers. He uses eating utensils well.

BEHAVIOUR, EMOTIONAL AND SOCIAL DEVELOPMENT
Zeke is a happy boy and he likes being at school. His anxiety level has reduced now that he is familiar with the people, environment and routines. With a great deal of encouragement and insistence he is very slowly beginning to show that he can accept boundaries and guidelines. This does depend on the activity and whether he's in a focused mood or preferring to seek self-stimulation activities e.g. spinning, sound-making, gazing, squeezing others, running away from adults or out

of a room. He would benefit from provision where there is regular input from a specialist Occupational Therapist, who can advise on a programme to address his sensory needs. He is at the early stages of trusting adults in the school and he is beginning to realise that he can make himself understood.

Zeke needs consistency, predictable routines and clear concrete guidelines at home and at school. He is responding well to the positive approach and the visual strategies used in the IRB. He needs a lot of adult support to build up his independent skills and to manage his own behaviour. Zeke is very unaware that other people have thoughts and feelings and prefers everything on his terms. He has little awareness of danger and will try to climb to look out of the windows in the classroom. This is a concern as Apple class is situated on the first floor. At school he cannot be left alone as he will run in and out of classrooms or when in the toilet he will climb, play with the taps and water or put his hands into the toilet.

ZEKE'S NEEDS:
- Opportunities to participate in learning, which address the main areas of impairment in autism - social understanding and behaviour, non-verbal communication, thinking and behaving flexibly and sensory perception and responses.
- Access to an augmentative communication system and the Picture Exchange Communication System to provide him with a means of initiating communication within a social context.

- To develop his ability to listen and follow adult direction.
- To develop and promote his spontaneous and functional communication skills and in so doing his awareness that he can make himself understood.
- To develop his waiting, listening, turn-taking and sharing skills when involved in individual and group work.
- To accept clear boundaries and guidelines within a consistent approach.
- To develop the ability to manage situations he may find stressful.
- To accept his play skills and his understanding and use of toys.

TESTIMONIES

Testimonies are usually given in church by Christians. This is when the persons speak candidly or openly about an experience which they believe God has helped them or provided for them.

TESTIMONY NUMBER 1.

After saying my prayer upon waking early one morning, I was led by the Holy Spirit to get back on my knees and say a special prayer for Zeke. I was obedient to the command from God so I got back down on my knees and prayed a special prayer for my son. At first I simply knelt down on my knees without uttering any words. Then I was led to pray this short prayer. 'Dear Lord Jesus, I don't know what lies ahead today for Zeke, only you know. But I am asking you to protect him from all harm and danger. I pray that you will send a special angel to protect him from harm whilst he's away from my care.'

As Zeke's behaviour had become unmanageable at lunch time when he joined the year one class, the arrangement requested of me from senior management was that I should pick him up at 12pm and bring him home to give him lunch, then bring him back to school at the end of the lunch time, when he would go straight to the classroom where he also would have his one-to-one support.

To my horror when I arrived at the school at 12pm to pick Zeke up I was met by the Head Teacher, who told me that Zeke had left the school and that staff were out and about looking for him. She reassured me that he had been found and that he was safe and well. I was numb because I couldn't believe how he could have left the premises despite having one-to-one support.

I instantly knew why God had wanted me to pray a special prayer for him. Zeke was eventually found sitting in the middle of the busy A10 dual carriageway. He was saved because a male teacher from a nearby school called Raglan saw him sitting in the road and managed to remove him and held him tight whilst they both sat on the nearby pavement. Fortunately those oncoming cars were stopped by the traffic lights.

I was informed by one of the witnesses that Zeke was heard singing loudly the following song. *'He'll be coming round the mountain when he comes. He'll be coming round the mountain when he comes. He'll be coming round the mountain, coming round the mountain, coming round the mountain when he comes. Singing yah, yah, yippee, yippee yah. Singing yah, yah, yippee, yippee yah. Singing yah, yah, yippee, yah yippee, yah yippee when he comes.'*

Apparently an angel had saved him from getting seriously hurt or killed. He held on to him as he was fighting and trying to get away from him. This incident confirmed to me that Zeke wasn't aware of danger. God also sent another angel, a driver who stretched his hand out of his car window to stop the oncoming traffic.

Can you imagine what could have happened to Zeke if he had safely crossed the road and went home and found that there was no one there to open the door for him to go in? I would usually pick him up for lunch and bring him back at the end of lunch play time.

I was concerned and wondered why it was not possible for Zeke to have a support worker supporting him during the lunch hour. Imagine the valuable social and speaking experience he could have had during this time. B.H.P. Primary School was totally responsible for Zeke's care when he went missing from the school unnoticed and was found at lunch time on the A10 dual carriageway. I removed Zeke from this school in that I felt the teachers were not acting responsibly enough and that the school was too close to the busy A10 dual carriageway.

At age six Zeke was transferred from BHP Primary School, where he began year one, and then continued his education at Bowes Primary School which had an Inclusion Base. In agreement with the Educational Psychologist, we felt his educational and communication needs would be met there. Zeke was also assigned to a mainstream class one year, below his chronological age within this school. It was a perfect arrangement for him.

During subjects like Physical Education (PE) Music, Dance, Art, and Drama, Zeke joined his mainstream class-peers. But when they were having the more academic subjects such as Science, Maths, English, History and Geography he would return to the Inclusion Base where he would engage in Independent Living activities such as cooking, making a shopping list, and going shopping, cleaning the classroom and washing up. In the Inclusion Base he would do basic number and money work.

TESTIMONY NUMBER 2

On the day of our imminent return from Zeke's first holiday to Jamaica when he was aged seven, something remarkable happened which I hope will remain in my memory for the rest of my life.

I had decided to arrive at the airport in Montego Bay much earlier than required so we could book our luggage in early and chill out in the departure lounge, and if necessary look around in the shops and do shopping for gifts to take back with us to England. After engaging in the latter activity I was feeling somewhat tired so I decided to sit down and relax on one of the comfortable chairs in the vicinity. Kelsey and Zeke were instructed to do the same. Zeke, as expected, did not share my sentiment so he decided to do a quick run about instead and big sister Kelsey had no other choice but to pursue a chase, following him for his safety and our sanity in case he went missing. Despite the quick speed of the escalator Zeke felt it would be quicker if he sprinted upwards on it, with Kelsey struggling to catch up with him. At this point I was helpless and could not join in with his sprinting. The only thing I could do was to pray quietly in my mind that Kelsey would catch up with him and that he would not be harmed in any way.

After ten minutes they were upstairs and out of my sight or view. My eyes caught the eyes of two elderly Afro-Caribbean women who were seated opposite me. They were looking at me with a sympathetic expression on their faces. One of these women asked me, 'Does your little boy behave like that all the time?' I sadly replied, 'Yes he does, especially if he thinks he won't get his own way'. This same lady commented, 'And he lives in England!?' I then added that, 'At school he has a learning support assistant'. The second woman then added, with a frown on her brow and a caring, screwed-up face, 'Your little boy is in a lot of pain, that's why he's behaving like that.' These two ladies looked at each other with piercing eyes and did not look at me again or utter another word to me.

When I looked to my left hand side I observed that Kelsey was holding Zeke by his collar and they were sitting on the seat closest to me, with Zeke holding a medium-sized shopping bag in his hand. My thoughts were clearly on the comment that the second woman had made; 'Your boy is in a lot of pain and that's why he's behaving like that.'

It was now four pm and it was being announced over the amplifier that it was time to commence boarding the plane. I remember leaving the women still seated because my children and I were in the cohort group required to commence boarding as announced over the amplifier. My thoughts were permanently pre-occupied with the comments that the two elderly women had made, but at the same time I felt relieved because I knew I had something very important to discuss with my general practitioner when I returned to London. 'I must get a second opinion on the previous MRI scan that was done on Zeke's head and upper body, over one year ago,' were the thoughts churning out over and over again in my head.

I kept looking behind me for the two women who were sitting close to me and speaking with me in the departure lounge but they were nowhere to be seen. I looked for them a few times when the plane was in the air but they were not seen. When we landed at Heathrow Airport I kept looking in different directions but they could not be seen. I simply wanted to tell them, 'Thank you,' and ask if they would allow for us to exchange telephone numbers. I simply concluded that they were my angels sent by God and once they had completed their assignment they disappeared.

CHAPTER 13:
PECS - Picture Exchange Communication System

" If you can't explain it simply, you don't understand it well enough" Albert Einstein

The Picture Exchange Communication System (PECS) was developed by Lori Frost MS, CCC/SLP and Dr Andrew Bondy in 1984. It was first used at the Delaware Programme to teach children with autism as a fast, self-initiating, functional communication system.

PECS begins with the exchange of simple pictures but progresses gradually to sentence structure. Many studies have confirmed that PECS helps people develop verbal language, decreases tantrums and odd behaviour and increases socialising with others.

Zeke was introduced to PECS at Bowes Primary School Inclusion Base. This communication system encouraged him to express his needs or wants by sequencing a series of pictures which are accompanied by single words or phrases. For example: I want water. This sentence strip would have the prepared words 'I want' followed by an arrow pointing to the picture of a cup of water. The word 'water' would also be written under this picture of the cup. At home we were encouraged through training by Zeke's class teacher to practice using PECS with Zeke.

We were initially given an A5 folder which had three horizontal Velcro strips glued to the outer cover. Inside this ring binder folder were three laminated sheets with another three horizontal strips attached to each sheet. On these strips were a carefully selected amount of words and picture cards as well as cards with short, two-word sentences such as: 'I want... toilet'; 'I like.... orange'. Some single words were also given. When Zeke wanted something he would fetch his folder and attempt to make his request by putting it on the sentence strip. In order to develop his speech I would get Zeke to try and read to me each of the sentences by repeating after me.

THE METHOD BELOW WAS ALSO USED TO DEVELOP ZEKE'S SPEECH AND COMMUNICATION.
BASIC MAKATON

Makaton was developed in the 1970s by Margaret Walker, MBE, as part of a research project. She was a speech and language therapist. Her assistants were Kathy Johnson and Tony Cornforth. The name Makaton originated by using the first syllables of each of the above names. Makaton is a unique programme which uses signs, symbols and speech to enable people to communicate. It supports the further development of communication skills such as attention, listening, comprehension and recall of taught words and expressions.

Alongside PECS, basic Makaton was used to help Zeke's speech to develop. Basic Makaton is the simplest form of sign language. This incorporates signing a word with the associated speech. For example, the sign for 'Thank you' would be accompanied by saying the words 'Thank you.' Simply put, it is a 'sign' and 'speak' method.

Zeke was encouraged to repeat after me each word that he had put on his sentence strip. Gradually Zeke would learn these words enough to be able to read them independently.

Zeke would also engage in a tailored literacy session to meet his particular needs. Zeke was granted an extra year at his lovely primary school which meant he was not transferred to a secondary school until the age of 12.

SOME SAMPLES OF ZEKE'S PRIMARY SCHOOL REPORTS
GENERAL INFORMATION
Zeke began attending the Inclusion Resource Base (IRB) on 15 September 2005 and is now in school full time. Zeke is supported within the Inclusion Resource Base (IRB) and is unable to access what is on offer in the mainstream part of the school. He integrates with his mainstream peers at playtime and at lunch time. He also attends a Key Stage 1 Music Assembly and some whole school assemblies. This report is based on two terms part-time attendance with 15 hours one-to-

one support provided by the Local Education Authority (LEA) until December 2005. This 15 hours support is now provided by the school because Zeke requires this support to keep him safe, keep him focused on tasks, prevent him from climbing through the window, from helping himself to resources, and from running out of the classroom or the playground.

There is a specialist teacher/manager, a specialist class teacher, one full-time teaching assistant, one part-time teaching assistant, one 1-1 teaching assistant support for Zeke and four other children in the IRB. The IRB is divided into clearly defined areas organised to be distraction-free, to enable a child to concentrate on the task at hand. The environment has a sense of space and order and work is organised to provide opportunities for learning functional activities using the Picture Exchange Communication System (PECS). Pupils are taught to initiate communication and to develop a social approach, within a social context. Pupils participate in both individual and group work in the IRB. There are opportunities for children in the IRB to be fully integrated into their mainstream classes and children from the mainstream join the IRB pupils for some lessons. Children from Key Stage 2 work with the IRB children as 'buddies' or role models.

RELEVANT HOME FACTORS

Zeke lives at home with his parents, older brother and sister. Mr and Mrs Sailsman are committed to ensuring that their son receives the best provision to meet his educational needs.

AUTISM – ONE FAMILY'S JOURNEY

They work collaboratively with professionals and are very supportive of the IRB/ Bowes Primary School. They have been informed that Zeke is working at a level below his peers and that the IRB may not be the most suitable provision for Zeke. Mrs Sailsman has informed me that she wants Zeke to remain in the IRB and in a mainstream school.

Zeke enjoys computer activities, ball games, bat and ball games, watching TV and videos, puzzles, music, spinning, squeezing other people, 'alphabet bus toy', comics, football stickers, football teams logo.

ZEKE'S AREAS OF NEEDS INCLUDE THE FOLLOWING:
- Opportunities to participate in learning, which address the main areas of impairment in autism - social understanding and behaviour, non-verbal and verbal communication, thinking and behaving flexibly and sensory perfection and responses.
- Access to augmentative communication system and the Picture Exchange Communication System to provide him with a means of initiating communication within a social context.
- To develop his ability to listen and follow adult direction.
- To build on social relationships with peers and adults.
- To develop and promote his spontaneous functional communication skills and in so doing his awareness that he can make himself understood.

- To develop his waiting, listening, turn taking and sharing skills when involved in individual and group work.
- To accept clear boundaries and guidelines within a consistent approach.
- To develop the ability to manage situations he may find stressful.
- To develop his play skills and his understanding and use of toys.
- To develop an understanding of socially appropriate and inappropriate behaviour at home and school.
- To develop coping strategies to deal with transitions, new environments, changes to routines, by developing his understanding of a surprise.
- To develop his ability to compromise and negotiate both at home and in school.
- To develop his ability to adjust to school expectations and routines.
- To develop the skills important for transition into mainstream education.
- To develop his self-help skills.

One criterion for full admission to the Inclusion Resource Base is that pupils should be able to spend a significant amount of time in the mainstream classroom, sometimes without support. At this stage Zeke has not been integrated into a mainstream classroom due to his current skills, the severity of his needs, the severity of his behaviour, his sensory integration needs, and his language and communication difficulties. He needs to develop sitting, looking and waiting skills, independently.

Zeke needs to develop his functional communication skills and his understanding and use of language. For example, responding to commands such as 'Come', 'Wait', 'Stop', on others' terms. He will need help in acquiring, comprehending, using language and generalising new skills in many environments and situations. He will need to be supported by teaching staff skilled in working with children with autism within a specialist setting. The opportunities for learning will need to be carefully structured and planned with finely graded sequences of objectives and targets specific to his needs.

Zeke has made great progress since attending the IRB. However, his needs would be better met in a school where he will have better access and opportunities to experience 'soft play', 'messy play', swimming, freedom to explore large playground equipment in a safe and secure environment and extensive access to a sensory curriculum.

The Bowes IRB for children with ASD has provided a structured environment and specialist teaching staff who have been able to address Zeke's needs. However, Zeke has needed full-time 1:1 support to be able to access what is on offer. The mainstream environment provides him with many challenges and he is functioning at a level below his Apple Class peers and his mainstream peers. He does not seek out the social rewards and company of his mainstream peers. Zeke is coping well in Bowes because he spent his time in the IRB and has the extra support of a 1:1 teaching assistant, which the school is now funding till the summer term. Without adult support we would not be able to meet Zeke's needs efficiently and effectively. He needs to be kept safe and on task as he does not have the understanding or prerequisite skills to focus on the salient aspects independently. Zeke needs a provision where the whole environment is safe and secure and there are no concerns when he runs off. Zeke would need 1:1 support to remain in the IRB.

ZEKES TRANSFER TO SECONDARY SCHOOL
When it was time for Zeke to be transferred to secondary school, it became very difficult to get him into a secondary school, even though the local authority would have funded a learning support worker to support him in the various classes. Unfortunately none of the mainstream schools offered him a place in their schools. Even the special schools for children with moderate learning difficulties did not offer him a place. As parents we concluded that there were two reasons why these schools would not offer him a place in their schools. These reasons are described below:

(i) Zeke had left his first primary school and was found sitting in the middle of the busy dual carriage road. We believe that secondary school managers were concerned that one day he may leave their school. They did not want to be held responsible should Zeke leave the school, unknown to staff, and get killed by a moving vehicle, snatched by an undesirable person or harmed in any other way.

(ii) I had reported the school to the Office for Standards in Education (OFSTED) because I strongly believed that it was a deliberate plan by Zeke's reception class teacher that he should leave the school premises. I believe so because I had expressed my disappointment at the lack of progress whilst in this teacher's class, during a recent annual review meeting. It was obvious to Zeke's father and me that basically, she no longer wanted Zeke in her class and she was finding a reason for him to be transferred to another school. In my opinion she nearly received a manslaughter conviction hanging on her head, and the revoking of her teacher's qualification, because Zeke had communicated to me that his teacher had told him to 'go home'.

Surprisingly the teacher's lack of care for him was not challenged because of the racist way in which the investigating police officer dealt with the incident. This police officer concluded that the teacher should not be blamed because Zeke only left the school because he knew that his mother was always at home. Surprisingly to me, this was not the case because I am at work most days, but I had to leave work each day to collect him from school at lunch times and bring him home to give him lunch, after which I would take him back to school for the afternoon session and then return again 2.5 hours later to pick him up at the end of the school day.

Based on the above assessments, Zeke's father and I had to accept a place at the only secondary school that would have him. This school was a special school for children with a diagnosis of autism and having severe learning and behaviour challenges.

The only reason why we agreed to a place for Zeke in that school was because we liked the high level of security in place. We felt that at least he would not be able to easily leave the premises. We also had the assurance that he had been equipped with enough learning skills to develop further. However, within one week of him being at his secondary school we noticed obvious changes in Zeke's behaviour towards us. He had started to lash out at us when we said 'No' to him. He had started to bite us and thump his father on the head quite hard, kicking at the door and causing the glass to break. We also noticed that he was not speaking as well as before. His handwriting changed to big bold letters on which there was a huge amount of over writing. He no longer had regular individual reading sessions.

My greatest concern was the discovery that for two years Zeke remained at the same P-levels. This is the grading system used to assess the development of children in special schools or for those with learning difficulties. Zeke remained on the same P- levels for two years in the following areas of learning: Reading, Writing, Spelling, Number Work and Science.

It became obvious to us that our son's academic education was being deliberately neglected at this special school. We discovered that 'independent living' training took precedence over his academic learning. This was the most important aspect of the children's learning within this special school.

It took me four years to realise and understand that when he began his education at this school that the staff had made the decision not to follow his updated Secondary Transfer Education Curriculum Planning. This secondary school did not follow on from the previous primary school and set targets . He was not making any progress as a result. When the Head Teacher was asked by an Independent Educational Psychologist why this had happened his explanation was that they have found that when children with autism leave a mainstream primary school to attend their special school, the levels they have been given are well below their assessment result.

Had we known that our son had been put back two years in his learning we would have attempted to establish the reason why, and maybe get an answer or an explanation. We would have most definitely appointed a tutor to help him with some kind of continuity in his learning, as recommended in his learning plan by his previous primary school.

My worries about Zeke's change of behaviour towards his parents were confirmed. Zeke's sudden change of behaviour showed that he was not happy at his secondary school. Or, were there other reasons for this change? I speculated that there was a lack of support and being excluded from mainstream-peers to which he was not accustomed.

THE INFORMATION BELOW WAS OBTAINED FROM ZEKE'S SECONDARY SCHOOL

1. Samples of Zeke's learning plans at various educational establishments
2. Summaries of Zeke's educational achievements
3. Areas of Learning

Personal Development - The area of Personal Development includes National Curriculum personal, social and health education (PSHE).

Citizenship and careers where appropriate - These include the ability to develop self-management and emotional control using strategies such as therapies, self-help, independence skills, attention and concentration skills, and health and safety awareness.

TARGET AGREED AT LAST REVIEW

1. To wait for up to 5 minutes appropriately for a desired activity with visual support initially, daily with 4 out of 5 successions (Achieved).
2. Summary of progress towards targets/Learning/ Achievement

Zeke is a very friendly young man who has continued to develop positive relationships with both the adults and pupils in his class. He has developed a good understanding of our class routines and he follows them on a daily basis with minimal prompting. Zeke's listening and concentration skills are getting better. He is able to sit quietly for longer periods of time and he's able to answer simple questions about our work.

Although Zeke's concentration has improved he does need an adult to sit beside him to help keep him focused on a task. When Zeke is engaged he will complete all his work. In PSHE we have covered the topics 'Organising an Event, Friendships and Making Choices.' Zeke has continued to make steady progress in PSHE.

Zeke has developed numerous independent skills such as washing up, drying and putting away cooking items after use, preparing his own breakfast every morning. Zeke participates in weekly practical life skills where he has experienced various skills.

The year 10 children take part in weekly ASDAN sessions, completing the transition challenge which is a modular course of five different areas. Zeke has completed the First Module called 'Knowing How' which involves independent living skills and working towards the next module 'Making Choices'.

Zeke's understanding of the topics covered has improved and with prompts he is able to recall what he has learnt in simple words. Zeke is beginning to develop his social skills.

Regular group choosing sessions within the classroom allow him to choose an activity and a friend to work together with. He is gaining an understanding of taking turns and playing games together. However, in order to progress further he must continue to apply himself fully to the tasks he is set.

THE TOPICS AND MODULES COVERED WERE THE FOLLOWING: ASDAN - Knowing How, Taking Part in a Charity Event, Class Rules, Friendship, Making Choices.

THE NEW TARGETS FOR NEXT YEAR INCLUDING STATEMENT SPECIFIC TASKS INCLUDED THE FOLLOWING:
- To take his time and eat his food slowly 80% of the time.
- To wait when asked by an adult at home time or when teacher is talking to parents 80% of the time.

The Area of Learning/ Behaviour/Attitude to learning included the following: The area of learning and attitude to learning includes any barriers to learning and how they are being addressed, as well as the development of emotional, social and behavioural skills to support cognition and learning skills.

SUMMARY OF PROGRESS TOWARDS TARGETS/LEARNING/ ACHIEVEMENT

Zeke contributed to the creation of his Class rules which has given him a sense of inclusion. These rules and expectations are clearly displayed within the classroom and referred to daily. He can identify that the consequence of his actions is a five minutes time-out. He does, however, need to develop his understanding of why these actions were inappropriate, which in turn will improve his behavioural skills. A reward system has been introduced into the classroom environment which Zeke fully understands. He receives stars for positive behaviour, throughout the school day. Zeke has on many occasions received the most stars throughout the day and has been rewarded at the end of school, allowing him to be more confident and develop his self-esteem.

At times Zeke experiences difficulty when asked to wait during lunch time and at the end of the school day. At these times with support he can remove himself from a stressful situation by going to the classroom and calm down. This helps Zeke to make choices and to cope when he finds himself in a stressful situation. The topics and modules covered were as follows: Class rules, Feelings, Helping Others and How to Behave in a Public Place.

The new targets for the next year including statements and specific targets were as follows: Zeke to sit and focus during lessons and Zeke to choose a friend to play a game with during choosing times and play times.

THE AREAS OF LEARNING FOR COMMUNICATION DEVELOPMENT WERE AS EXPLAINED AS FOLLOWS:
The area of communication development includes National Curriculum English literacy and speech, language and communication skills, supported by the speech and language therapists. The development of autism-specific communication strategies will be used to support everyday interactions such as Intensive Interaction and Dance Write.

THE TARGETS AGREED AT LAST REVIEW WERE AS FOLLOWS:

- To develop Zeke's language so that he is able to answer a question or comment on what he can see in each lesson using a person + action or action + object place sentences with visual support, daily with 3/5 success. (Partly achieved)
- To read a small paragraph and answer questions in a structured situation with support from PECS initially, daily with 3/5 success. (Target changed by Speech Therapist)

THE SUMMARY OF PROGRESS TOWARDS TARGETS/LEARNING/ ACHIEVEMENTS WERE EXPLAINED AS FOLLOWS:

Zeke has continued to make steady progress in literacy this year. He is able to communicate his thoughts and wants through symbols and speech. He is able to answer using short sentences, including key words used within a session. Zeke is beginning to remember the characters' names, where the story takes place and key elements of the plot. When questioned following a story or a discussion Zeke can answer simple questions and he is beginning to use a more varied vocabulary provided he has access to PECS pictorial prompts. At times Zeke needs to be encouraged, as he does not always volunteer to participate. This year in literacy we have been working on helping Zeke to develop his language, comprehension skills and extending vocabulary knowledge. Zeke is responding well to the colour coded text where he has to answer simple 'Who' questions. Zeke enjoyed reading *Charlie and the Chocolate Factory* and *Jack and the Beanstalk* stories.

Zeke has a firm pincer grip and his handwriting has improved. His letters are not always consistent in size but they are formed correctly. Zeke's writing is neat and legible and when focused he works really well. Zeke can copy text during writing activities and complete sentences providing he has the missing words but will request support to construct his own sentences. As his speech and language skills continue to improve he will be able to construct longer and more accurate sentences.

Zeke is continuing to develop his reading skills although at times he can be quite hesitant and lacks confidence. He needs to develop his phonic awareness further so that he can apply it to deciphering and reading unknown words. Zeke needs to gain confidence and use his phonic knowledge further so that he spells more words independently.

THE TOPICS AND MODULES COVERED WERE AS FOLLOWS:
ASDAN - Knowing How, Book Study, Poems and Media- Newspaper, Stories, AQA - Beginning to recognise and use signs for places.

THE NEW TARGETS FOR NEXT YEAR INCLUDING STATEMENT SPECIFIC TARGETS WERE AS FOLLOWS:
Zeke to express likes and dislikes verbally with visual support in structured situations 4 times per week with 3/5 success. Zeke to be able to understand WH- questions, (who, what, where, when) relating topic to work and weekend news or recent event; 80% of the time.

The area of fine and gross motor skills includes National Curriculum PE, Swimming and Leisure where appropriate. This will also include any occupational therapy including the development of sensory integration.

THE TOPIC COVERED WERE AS FOLLOWS:
Gymnastics, Dance and Games
Zeke was working on travelling and balancing in gymnastics before Christmas. He was moving around the gym floor in various ways - rolling, jumping, crawling, hopping, plus holding his body in different balance positions. His focus was to alternate between travelling and balancing, creating his own sequence and transferring his body weight in a controlled and safe manner.

Zeke worked through the objectives (he paired verbal and physical gestures), and carried out a short, but clear routine. The theme was 'Laugh a minute', humorous gestures were explored and peer interactions were encouraged throughout.

The focus for the term was different size and direction, plus mirroring/shadowing and working in a small group. Fitness and health is an ongoing focus.

Zeke reacts well to repetition and his personal focus is to participate with less verbal prompting.

In regards to Inclusion the following explanation was given:
Zeke has had the opportunity to join groups of pupils from other classes within the department for music, dance and drumming.

Zeke's Class will have the opportunity to visit the local primary school for various projects, and will continue to create opportunities to share activities within the local community too. There will also be opportunities for Zeke to take part in work experience in the charity shop.

Although this secondary school had a sixth form college attached to it, we became so disillusioned with the school that at the age of 16 we had Zeke transferred to an outer borough sixth form college, where he remained for three years until the age of 19 in July 2018.

Having been at this sixth form college Zeke made steady progress. His teachers and support workers have been very supportive, respectful and honest with us concerning his progress. This working relationship has enabled us to do more with Zeke at home. We filled the gaps that had not been sufficiently met in the classroom, such as daily 1-1 reading sessions with one of his parents.

CHAPTER 14:
Lack of support from a social worker-representative

"Life is about making a contribution, not about being popular and fitting in" Rudy Simone

Let's imagine the scenario of a social worker being appointed by the Local Education Authority to attend the annual review of a child with learning difficulties. The situation is this: a female social worker was appointed to Zeke and her main duty was to accompany my husband and me to Zeke's annual review meeting. Zeke had turned five years old, and had to be transferred from Reception class to Year One. We were appointed a social worker to help to prepare us for the interview and Statement of Special Needs application for an autistic child. This application is now called an Education Health Care Plan (EHCP).

In our understanding her main role was to help us understand the process and significance of a formal diagnosis of autism. When I began to ask questions at this meeting in order to get clarity around the 'pros and cons' of a child receiving a Statement of Special Needs, our appointed social worker appeared to be antagonistic towards me because I was asking questions for some clarity.

As far as she was concerned, the senior management decision was what counts and their plan towards the future of our son's education and care should not be questioned. Instead we should accept, even though we did not understand the possible outcome of, their decisions. When I continued to ask questions that were necessary to us, surprisingly this social worker abruptly got up from her chair and asked that she be excused to leave, and she simply left without even looking at us parents. At this time I was debating over our choice of in-class support worker from the two ladies who were currently doing a job share in their role as Zeke's in-class support worker.

That was the last we saw and heard from that appointed social worker. I thought that she would have contacted me afterwards to discuss the outcome of the meeting but she never did.

After this encounter we were never appointed another representative to accompany us to annual reviews again, so we were left to face all challenges and bureaucratic situations on our own.

When the Head Teacher and the Special Educational Needs Co-Ordinator (SENCO) of the school were debating that they would prefer that Zeke is supported by one of their permanent support workers, our social worker commented that I should adhere to the school's decision because at least they were providing a support worker for him.

The other in-class support worker was independent of the school and as a result she was discharged, and the school's permanent support worker was chosen, who was not as competent as the independent support worker. However, the independent support worker was professional enough to provide me with some useful learning tools to work on with Zeke within the home. This wonderful lady gave me the drive and determination to persevere with Zeke. She advised me to read to Zeke for a few minutes every day, which I did, even until today, which Zeke enjoys.

CHAPTER 15:
Career, profession and my life postponed

"I"d rather regret the risk that didn't work out than the chances I didn't take at all." Simone Biles

At age 55 I made the conscious decision that I should remain at home and become the main carer for my son. I basically came to a turning point in my life where I began thinking about what is best for Zeke. I had been living in hope that by the age of twelve Zeke's speech would have developed to near normal for his age. That unfortunately did not happen so I decided that I needed to make myself more available to him to ensure that he was getting as much as possible from the secondary school that he was attending.

I also felt that I had a lot more to offer to him than what I was offering to him while I was managing my private childcare centre in the London borough of Haringey. His dietary needs also needed to be given more consideration as in addition to Autism (ASD), he also had Attention Deficit Hyperactive Disorder (ADHD). I closed down my daycare centre in May

2013 and more or less opted for a life of meditation.

Mentally I discovered I was exhausted. Physically I was tired and socially I had no true friends and no supportive relatives. My husband and I were constantly at each other's throats. Our first and second born became almost absent from the home and rarely sat and ate meals with us. Our lives completely revolved around Zeke, who seemed very unhappy with life and everyone around him. I felt that this atmosphere needed to change and that the only person who could do that was the mother of the home, which happened to be me.

The first thing I changed was our cooking and eating habits. Breakfast time remained the same as my family members prefer cereals, so I simply encouraged everyone to sit at the table and eat their individual cereal together. My husband seemed to enjoy organising breakfast time so I encouraged him to continue to do so while I remained in the background, attempting to motivate my family members to engage in conversation with each other as 'role models' for Zeke's speech development.

My husband and I decided that we would take turns taking Zeke to school while I collected him in the evenings. Once the rest of my family were out and about getting on with their daily activities I would remain at home engaged in activities such as cleaning, cooking and ironing. Previously I had a lovely lady who would visit the home twice weekly to do my cleaning and ironing. Her help could no longer be afforded and I was content in taking on those chores myself. In between these chores I would make time to put my feet up and have a rest. The most enjoyable chore was cooking the evening meals. I would start cooking the evening meals at 12pm and finish at 2pm. This would allow me to leave home at 2.30pm in order to arrive at Zeke's secondary school on time to pick him up at 3pm.

I noticed that Zeke was looking happier and that he was initiating conversation more with me and the rest of his family members. Within two weeks I noticed a positive drastic change in the persona of all my family members. Everyone seemed happier, my first and second born were staying in more at home. My first born, a daughter, was making a real effort to assist me with the domestic chores. Generally our mother-daughter relationship was rekindled. My second born, a son, was speaking more with his father and me. My husband was making a real effort to talk to me in a pleasant way and complementing me on the meals l had prepared for the family. He was even making suggestions that we should have a night out while our two oldest children remained at home to watch Zeke, at least until we returned home after our outing.

After six weeks at home we began to struggle financially much more than before. I had an idea to make a phone call to our local 'Carers centre' and I was put through to a lovely lady called Bridget. Bridget introduced herself as the Carers' benefits advisor. By the end of our conversation an appointment was booked for me to see her to establish the type of benefits I might be eligible to receive being the main carer of my son, who has a diagnosis of autism. Bridget completed all the necessary benefits paperwork and asked me to sign and date them. Within two weeks I received an email stating my entitlements and the total amount I would receive four-weekly. £245.00 was the amount awarded. It was explained that with that amount, if I wished to work I could work a maximum of 16 hours per week without affecting my benefit.

I decided that I wanted to work on a Saturday when my other family members were mostly at home. So I decided to gain some experience in the work involved at 'Child Contact Centres'. In the meantime I updated my CV and submitted it to an organisation that outsourced experienced workers to work in 'supervisory' to 'Accessed Child Contact Centres' across London. I held this position for six consecutive Saturdays but soon found it exhausting as I was based in Brixton. Staff at this particular centre were noticeably hostile towards each other and management was constantly paying my wages late. During this time I continued in my voluntary role, working between two different contact centres in my home borough for the duration of twelve months.

I later decided that I would return to the classroom as a Learning Support Worker for two days per week. I contacted my local borough which informs residents of job vacancies as they arise. I was accepted and was placed on the relief staff register. The first school in which I was placed was situated in an affluent area where I was appointed to support a Year Six girl with ASD diagnosis, who was adorable. I did not, however, like the attitude of one particular girl in the class, who was rude and very disrespectful towards me.

On one occasion I attempted to assist her to organise her tray as she appeared to be struggling to complete the task. After I had completed the summer term in that classroom I decided that I did not wish to return to that particular school. However, when I was asked to support a Year Five boy with mild autism, whom I knew through the school's lunch time club that I had previously supported, I willingly accepted this role.

To my horror I was not aware that I was about to experience my first obvious racism from the class teacher, a young woman in her early thirties. This experience confirmed to me that racism still exists and that the sooner I leave that particular school the happier I'll be.

The next school I was placed in was within two miles of the first one but the racism was similar, although it came from the Teaching Assistant in the Reception class. Again, I decided that I would not return to that school.

The third school I was placed in was situated in the most deprived area of the borough, about three miles from the second school and five miles from the first. It wasn't racism on this instance.

The classroom assistant, whose job was to support the whole class, then intentionally took on my role as 1-1 support worker for a Somalian boy who had mild autism. I felt undermined as I was assigned as a 1-1 support worker but was prevented from doing this role because the classroom assistant was intentionally spending time with the one child that had autism and not supporting the whole class anymore. She had switched her role to mine, where she instantly became 1-1 support worker to the boy who I was placed in that class to support.

She had left me with no choice but to become the classroom assistant. This was not my job. It was my job to support the child who had autism. The class teacher did not appear to be aware that this change of role by her classroom assistant had taken place. The staff and children within the entire school were from multicultural backgrounds, which I greatly admired.

This attitude I can cope with, because I could have asserted myself and said 'No,' but I decided that I also did not wish to return to that school. Currently on a number of occasions I'm being asked to offer learning support in three lovely schools and so far the experience and attitude from staff towards me are encouraging. I decided that I will therefore accept requests to engage in support work within these particular schools only. Coupled with work within these schools, I am writing my second book. I will also engage in activities to develop my autism business as well as promote and market my first book, called 'She caused the lightning to strike.'

CHAPTER 16:
Fears after the diagnosis of autism in my son

"My future depends mostly upon myself." Paul Robeson

My biggest fear following Zeke's diagnosis with ASD was how I would be perceived and received in the black community and how he would be received by his cousins and other mainstream or neuro-typical peer groups. As a result I decided that I would not quickly disclose this diagnosis to anyone closest to me. My plan was that I would, however, be honest if they did show concerns about his development or if they asked questions.

Eighty-year-old Pastor Charles MacFarlane, who was the pastor of the church which we attended, made a request to the members of the church in my local borough that they should assist us as much as possible with the care of Zeke. But no member except his ailing widow came forward to support us on a few occasions. She did so in ways that was effective and helpful. Missionary Daphne Macfarlane, with all her good intentions to support Zeke and me, was unable to do so due to ill health. In all good intentions she was unable to give much support. We thanked her very much for her help.

Instead of helping the family by offering support to Zeke, some of the members were inclined to be putting demands on my husband to commit more of his time to taking on duties in the church whilst leaving me at home to take care of Zeke alone, as well as making myself available to our two older children. I concluded that they were clearly ignorant of the behaviour and needs of a child who has autism. I was left with no further option but to find another church where the leaders as well as the members were supportive to the needs of Zeke, by now a teenager.

Lincoln Road Chapel was our second chosen church. To start with, we discovered that there was a Friday youth club that was willing to integrate youths with learning difficulties with support into their sessions. We also discovered that Zeke would be integrated into the Sunday services, again with support. As a result Zephie, my husband and I decided to accept the 'Right Hand of Fellowship' at our new church, and after six years we have become fully fledged members of the church. I did attempt to become involved in their Babies and toddlers group but had experience of racism from a young mother who is not a member of the church. Another mother who was holding a baby while his mother joined the queue to get refreshment. This mother had asked me to hold the baby so that she could also go and get refreshment. When the mother of the baby who by now had got her refreshment and was seated comfortably and talking with someone, but noticed who was holding her baby, she stormed over towards me and shouted at me, 'give me my baby and quickly took her baby then sat down beside me leaving one chair gap. She then said 'it looks like you've forgotten something! I was so shocked that I could not utter a word in my defence. For that reason I decided to withdraw myself completely from the volunteer role and opted for staying at home instead.

MEDICATION

At the age of twelve Zeke's newly assigned paediatrician at the hospital made a decision for Zeke to be put on a medication called CONCERTA. Concerta medication is used to treat 'Attention deficit disorder' (ADHD or ADD). It is a central nervous system stimulant which contains 'methylphenidate'. This medication is used to activate the speech and language centre of the brain. Zeke remained on this medication for three years until I decided that it was doing him more harm than good.

    The instruction given by the paediatrician in regards to how it should have been administered to him was that he was to take one tablet after a full breakfast from Monday to Friday and that he should not take any on Saturday and Sunday. I was informed by his teacher that at school Zeke was a model student, meaning he did as he was asked and followed instructions very carefully. However, at home over the weekend he would become very angry, which would result in violence towards us, his parents.

When I made a complaint to his teacher who also happened to be the Special education needs coordinator (SENCO) of the school with the belief that they would give us support and possibly equip us with skills to manage his behaviour, the SENCO decided to refer me to the school's psychiatrist because she felt I was the problem, as Zeke did not display such behaviour at school.

I was discharged from the psychiatrist clinic at the end of my first visit as he disagreed with the SENCO's assessment of me. I began to read up more about the Concerta medication. I discovered that the CONCERTA SUPPRESSES AGGRESSIVE BEHAVIOUR. During this time his named teacher, the most efficient of all the teachers in the entire school, informed us that Zeke was not speaking to the children or staff.

I relayed this information to the hospital paediatrician who concluded that the CONCERTA seemed to be not only suppressing his aggressive behaviour but it was also supressing his expressive speech. The paediatrician decided that it was time he was taken off the CONCERTA medication. My fears were confirmed, the CONCERTA medication was responsible for a reduction of Zeke's speech. Within three days of not taking the Concerta, Zeke gradually stopped lashing out at us and was making a real effort to communicate verbally to us.

During this same period I discovered that Zeke's teachers were not following the recommended procedure in the end of primary school HCP (Individual Healthcare Plan). In fact, they were using a plan which was three years out of date. This particular plan was for when he was nine years old, instead of using the one prepared at age twelve. This latter plan would have been prepared for when he left primary school to commence his secondary education.

Zeke was obviously discriminated against by SENCO and the Head Teacher of his secondary specialist school because they appeared to have deliberately held him back in his learning. Instead of building onto the previous skills which he had already learnt they made him repeat them. These activities were mainly concerned with gross and fine motor skills development. By age sixteen years he had developed beautiful looking handwriting. He was learning new techniques in playing football with enthusiasm.

He also developed a tremendous interest in playing basketball and tennis. However, his speaking and reading skills were almost totally neglected. Had the secondary school teacher followed his correct or current Individual Learning Plan, regardless of being in a disruptive classroom, his speech would have developed further.

Once I discovered the injustices on Zeke I then decided that I should remove him from that particular school and enrol him in an inclusive Sixth Form College where he could have a fresh start. Hence, we were then able to secure a place for him at an outer borough Sixth Form College. The first week was unsettling for Zeke, but once he was transferred to the ICT course from the Catering course which he was initially placed on, he settled down very quickly. His new teachers and support staff informed me that he was very talkative and helpful to his peers when they needed support on the computer.

After two years of being at this Sixth Form College I received lots of positive feedback about him. I was told that he was the brightest in his class. His teachers felt happy with his progress, saying he would be able to hold down a skilled full-time job. As a result he has been moved to a class of higher functioning children with the possibility of having some lessons with a group of mainstream students.

Zeke is now entering his third and final year at Sixth Form College. His prospects look brighter and we're hoping that in one year's time he will embark onto a three-year course which will shape his future for a successful work life and career. Zeke has maintained that he would like to study Computers, Art and Sports at college. So we're hoping that he will secure a course which will enable him to develop further in these subjects, commencing in September 2018.

The final question many people may ask is, 'Will Zeke find true love with a young lady?' Will he find a secure paid employment ?','Will he settle down, get married and have children?' My answer to these questions is that I cannot see any reasons why these shouldn't happen.

Since starting at the Sixth Form College at age sixteen Zeke has demonstrated an interest in using his IPAD computer and mobile phone to do short videos of people as they passed by in front of our house. However, he seems to be more focused on the little boy who lives across our road, directly opposite our house, who also has autism. After recording these short film clips he organises them in different ways and watches them as if he is watching a film on the television. He will make comments about them in a pleasant way. At times he will share the joke with us and when asked, 'What he's laughing about?' we will be told by him to 'Go away'.

I have no doubt in my mind that Zeke will one day find love. He is clearly attracted to the opposite gender as he likes to be in the company of girls in his age group. He talks passionately about two girls in his class and mentions when they're off sick from college. He asks if he could buy birthday cards for them and scribbles their names regularly on his notepad.

I do expect one day he will be heartbroken by a few girls because of the way that he may feel about them. But they might not feel the same way about him. I'm hoping that he will be mentally strong enough to cope with these rejections, and simply be able to move on with his life and hold on to his belief and trust in his God Lord Jesus, whom I know he loves and admires.

In terms of Zeke starting and developing an intimate relationship, and maintaining one, I'm reasonably confident that this will happen. But for this relationship to be successful this young lady will need to have similar needs as he. Or she will need to have a very high level of knowledge of the needs of a person with autism.

In terms of raising his own children, Zeke will need to have completed a tailored course in childcare and have completed work experience where he's observed and have participated in caring for newborn babies and very young children. Hopefully, he will marry a lady who has supportive parents and extended families. With these in place, she would have had first-hand experience of caring for babies, to the extent where she will be able to offer guidance to Zeke when he appears to be lacking the skills to effectively care for a baby.

I pray that God will give us the opportunity to be alive until he becomes a fully grown man. I also pray that his relationship with his older brother and sister, their spouses, their children, and their friends will remain strong. I pray that God will also bless Zeke with genuine, trusted friends and work colleagues that will treat him like a true friend or relative. I also pray that he will have at least two hobbies that he loves and enjoys so much that he will simply bury himself in them, especially when faced with difficult times, particularly when friends and families can't be found.

EMPLOYABILITY, INTIMATE RELATIONSHIP AND RAISING HIS OWN CHILDREN

I have a high level of confidence that Zeke will be able to hold down a job and perform extremely well in the role that has been assigned for him. Zeke has expressed interest in all sports. Since the age of twelve he has told his parents that when he becomes a man he would like to become a 'sports writer of books.' Since the age of three he has been able to accurately recognise and give the names of popular football clubs as well as the names of each player. He can also recognise and read the make and model of all cars he sees.

Zeke could recognise the model and make of a car from a distance. Some of them were foreign cars. I felt so proud of Zeke's quick observation and attention to detail. There won't be an issue around timing and punctuality with Zeke in his employment. Due to the fact that Zeke is very meticulous in what he does, things have to be done precisely and accurately for Zeke, no short cuts. As a result his performance will be of a very high standard. He also shows a passion for dancing and singing.

During the summer holidays, Zeke's personality changed almost overnight. He developed a comical streak, cracking jokes and laughing hilariously. The boy across the road from our house, whom I mentioned earlier, also has a diagnosis of autism. Zeke would sit and watch his daily movements outside and simply make fun of him. He would say things like 'Tommy wakes up at 4 o'clock. Tommy going to my old school,' which is not true. He says all this in a fit of laughter. When I tell him that I will be taking him to that same school again, he comically begs and says, 'No, No.'

UNCERTAINTY OF WHETHER AUTISM RUNS IN MY FAMILY AS WELL AS ZEKE'S FATHER'S FAMILY.

I have always believed that autism is not genetic and that it does not run in my family. Also deep down in my mind, I have reasons to believe that autism ran in Zeke's father's side of the family. In reflection on this matter, there is a known fact that from both sides of my parents' families there have been mostly male relatives, as close as uncles who have moved away from the region in which they were born in Jamaica to set up homes in other regions of Jamaica, far away, and have never returned to visit their relatives.

The relatives they left behind would at times go to visit them but they never reciprocated. Most were married and had children of their own. In some cases they had fathered so many children that financially they were unable to send them to school, so some of their children were given away to other families who would send them to school and use them as helpers in their home and on the farm. Most of these male children would engage in work involving working on the farm and taking care of animals. There have been similar cases in Zeke's father's side of his family, where, male relatives were given away to other families far away from their blood relatives.

In 1994 my husband, our two older children and I went on holiday to Jamaica specifically to visit my much-loved ailing mother. During this time we had the opportunity to visit some relatives I had not met before who were living in the parishes of Clarendon and St Thomas, which happen to be over 80 miles away from St Elizabeth, their parish of origin. In Clarendon, I firstly met two adult male second cousins, Nathan and Ansell. There was something unusual about their behaviour and from the moment I set eyes on them, I became concerned. In my mind, I wondered why they were portraying such unusual behaviour. At first, they appeared to be shy and lack in confidence to be around strangers, even though their brother Leonard, who had relocated from England and was living with them, had introduced us, saying that we were cousins.

Ansell, the older of the two men, was about fifty years old and he was very talkative and friendly. However, his speech was not directed at us because he was not making eye contact with any of the six people looking at him and listening to him. The topic he was talking about made sense but I did not feel comfortable to engage in his conversation. The others in our company also did not make any comment, they only listened to him until he had stopped talking.

Nathan, the younger, who was about 43 years old, did not utter a word to anyone. He simply stood around with an absent look in his eyes and an expressionless face and showed no emotion. He appeared to be withdrawn to me, while Ansell appeared to be hyperactive and engaged. Their behaviour resembled someone who could have Asperger's or autism. But looking back, I began to believe that they were on the autistic spectrum.

Two years later in 1996 my siblings and I, with my immediate family, returned to Jamaica for the memorial service of our well-loved mother who had passed away previously in 1995. After this event had taken place we had the opportunity to visit some relatives in St Thomas. To be honest, I was really shocked and embarrassed to see the living conditions of this particular female relative of mine. Yes, she was living in a small two bedroom dilapidated house with her elderly husband, a teenage daughter, who was the mother of a toddler and her youngest son who was in his early twenties.

My attention was instantly drawn to this handsome young man with a clean and well-kept appearance. His mother was clearly happy to see us and gladly called him over to where we were standing in the middle of the yard, surrounded by fruit trees. He gladly came towards me first. He shook hands with me while muttering incoherent words. I was clearly distraught by this revelation, because it was clearly obvious he was unable to communicate verbally. My heart sank into my chest and I felt sad. I said quietly to his mother, my first cousin Daphne, 'What's wrong with him?' She replied that he was 'deaf and dumb'.

Nevertheless, he was happy to pick up a long pole stick from the ground and began picking coconuts from the tree. Afterwards he indicated by hand gestures and some muttering and incoherent speech that they were for us. My cousin Daphne proceeded to volunteer information about him. She said that 'he was a very clever boy' and that 'he gets picked up by a school bus to go to a special school in Kingston, where he has learnt sign language and other subjects'. However, it wasn't until 2018 when I had a conversation with his eldest sibling that I was told that he was diagnosed with autism.

I concluded in my mind that relatives should be in regular contact, not only as financial support for each other but to be aware that certain medical conditions run in families.

In regards to my husband's family, particularly his mother's side of the family, there are classic cases of Asperger's amongst them. This manifests itself in them speaking and acting in ways which could be seen as anti-social behaviour. Basically, many of them will speak negative things about other people in their company without giving consideration to the hurtful impact on the feelings of their victims.

CHAPTER 17:
Zeke's transition to adulthood

"There needs to be a lot more emphasis on what a child can do instead of what he cannot do." **Temple Grandin**

At the age of 16-19 Zeke developed a habit of using every opportunity he got to leave the family home. These were very worrying times for his father and me. The first time this happened was between 10am and 11am in February 2017. Zeke managed to force open the downstairs living room window and had climbed out of the window while his father was out doing the weekly shopping and I was resting upstairs. Luckily, I was able to spot this early enough so I went looking for him and I found him at the local grocery store. I told him off and then explained to him that he could get snatched by a stranger. He replied, 'Sorry, Mummy,' and promised, 'I won't do it again.'

The second occasion that Zeke left the house without anyone noticing was on a Sunday between 8.30am and 9.30 am, during the Easter holidays in April 2017. His father had gone to Birmingham in the Midlands to visit his elderly father. Again, Zeke had forced the living room window open and had escaped. This time I was upstairs having a nap in my bedroom.

As soon as I realised that he had left the house, I telephoned 999 and reported the incident to the police. The police found him walking along the busy main road near our home. He was carrying his scooter under his arm and a carrier bag of groceries in his hand. The police stopped the car and asked him his name. He gave them his full name. They told him that I was at home worrying about him so he should get into the car and they would take him home. The police informed me that Zeke did not fuss and that he willingly sat in the back passenger seat of their car and was driven home.

I was standing at the gate of our house waiting; it was such a relief when I saw the police car pulling up outside my gate and noticed that they had found him. As soon as he came out of the car, he threw himself into my arms and apologised saying, "Sorry, Mummy." One of the woman police officers handed his bag of groceries to him and said, 'Here's your groceries, Zeke,' while the other police officer handed his scooter back to him. Inside his bag of groceries were an extra large sliced white loaf of bread and a large box of sugar-coated cornflakes cereal. These two items were not usually included on our grocery list due to the high calories and sugar content.

At this point one of the police officers explained that he'd seen young people in his age group travelling about in the community independently, and in small groups, and he wanted to be able to do the same. The other police officer added that he didn't want to be travelling around with his mum and dad all the time. The police officers were in support of us getting a 'buddy friend' of similar age to him, who could accompany him to the shops and to the park. I followed up on their suggestion by employing a young man from our church who was four months Zeke's junior.

This young man became Zeke's support worker in February 2017, and continued on a regular basis during school holidays and on Saturdays. In mid- May 2017, another young man four years Zeke's senior was appointed to replace the above, as a permanent part-time support worker for him.

The third time that Zeke left the house without anyone knowing was between 2pm and 3pm in May 2017. He had yet again forced the window of the living room open and this time it was broken and could not easily be fixed. It was a Saturday and fortunately his father was not at work, but had briefly left the house, and I was busy in the kitchen. When I could not see him I realised that he had left the house.

I then dialled 999 and reported him missing to the police as I'd been instructed to do by the police, since the first time he had left the house without anyone knowing. I next called his dad on his mobile and he said that he would be going to Edmonton Green shopping centre to look for him. This is a place that Zeke frequently went shopping with his dad, during the daytime, particularly during the school holidays. Thankfully, his dad found him in JD Sports shop looking at sportswear.

The fourth time that Zeke went missing was between 3pm and 4pm on a Saturday in August 2017. On this occasion he had left the family home fully clothed but wearing his socks and no shoes. The window and front door remained locked; the back door of the house was closed, but not locked. Before phoning 999 I searched the shed in the back garden, the neighbourhood and visited the local park which happened to be Ponders End Park. I asked a group of Afro-Caribbean youths if they had seen him. They said that they had seen him and that he was not wearing any shoes, only his socks. Another group of men at the barber shop at the corner of Lincoln Road said he was seen walking towards ASDA. Not only did I walk down to Ponders End train station in search of Zeke but I also went into ASDA to look for him. Unfortunately, he had gone much further away than the direction that had been given to me by the men who had told me that they'd seen him. In a panic, I dialled 999 and reported him missing then I returned home, hoping he had returned home on his own.

An hour had elapsed and it was getting dark, and Zeke had not been found. I feared for his safety and his life. I then began to pray for his safe return. When our house phone rang, it was the police. He had been found. Within fifteen minutes a police van was pulled up outside of my front door, but I could not see Zeke in the van. To my surprise one of the policemen went to the back of the van and opened that door. I quickly moved towards the door, where I saw Zeke sitting down and it suddenly dawned on me that he had travelled in the space where any suspected criminal would have been placed after being arrested. My spirit grieved. I then vowed to myself that he would never get treated in that way again. I honestly expected to see him sitting in the rear visible passenger seat.

The two policemen followed Zeke and me into the house, where they explained where and how he had been found. Afterwards they completed their paperwork and documentation. Thankfully, the shop keeper of the shop in Edmonton Green which he had entered had telephoned the police. This shop keeper had explained to the police that, 'A young man was in his shop rummaging amongst the magazines and that he's not wearing shoes, only socks, and appears to be ill.' In the presence of the police, again, I explained the danger to Zeke of him being out alone. He stroked my right arm with tears in his eyes and said, 'Sorry, Mummy, won't do it again.' Then he left the living room and went up to his bedroom.

The fifth time that Zeke left the house unknown to me was between 4pm and 5pm on 22 December 2017. On this occasion his dad was at work and I was upstairs having a nap. To my surprise I could feel a cold draft of wind blowing on my face as I slept in my bed upstairs. I quickly jumped off my bed and ran downstairs, where I found the front door of the house ajar.

I went outside and stood at the gate to our house, looking up and then down the road, but Zeke could not be seen. I left the door open and went back inside, where I called loudly, 'Zeke! Zeke!' I ran through the kitchen and checked the back door; it was locked. I said to myself, 'It looks like that boy has left the house again.' I continued checking all the rooms, cupboards, wardrobe in his bedroom and under his bed but Zeke clearly was not in the house. I walked to the top of our road, then to the bottom of our road. I then went into the two corner shops nearest to our home but Zeke was nowhere to be found.

None of the people walking along in our neighbourhood that I had spoken to about him having gone missing had seen him. I could not do anything more but dial 999 and report him missing to the police. By now thirty minutes had passed and it was getting dark. I feared for his safety and for his life. I was visited by three policemen, and after speaking to me for approximately ten minutes I was told that they were going to the local parks to look for him.

To my surprise, while still standing outside at the gate to our home, I heard footsteps of someone running which was coming from the end of our road at the side road nearest to our road. It was Zeke running towards me, with his rucksack on his back and a Nando's brown paper bag in his left hand. I waited at the gate for him but did not utter a word to him until he met with me at the gate. He was almost breathless and panting for breath. I simply said, 'Oh, Zeke, where were you? The police are out looking for you.' Zeke replied, 'Ponders End Retail Park.' Instantly I had a flash back.

I remembered that in December 2016, a few days before Christmas, Zeke had escaped from the holiday 'Teen scheme' in Southgate and was found by the project staff in a local charity shop. Enough said on this scenario.

Zeke initiated going inside our house while I remained outside. I then telephoned the number I had been previously given by the police squad room to use, if he returned before the police had found him. I quickly reported to the officer that he had returned home on his own.

While waiting for the three policemen to return, I checked inside the Nando's brown bag that he had left on the coffee table in the living room. I found three pairs of sports socks which were clearly marked 'Sport's Direct'. I then found in this Nando's bag two unopened drinking straws. I then proceeded to check his rucksack which he had left on the floor, leaning on the side of the coffee table before going upstairs to his bedroom, but nothing else was found. I thanked God in my mind that there was nothing else found. I noted that he was clearly prepared for his trip because inside this rucksack I found his wallet, his oyster card and his key to the front door of the house.

Within fifteen minutes the policemen were at our front door. I quickly opened the door and started apologising for wasting police time. One of them interrupted by saying, 'Thanks for notifying the department promptly.' He went on to say, 'As soon as the head office got your call we were contacted straight away so, no time was wasted.'

In the autumn of 2017, when Zeke had turned 18, his father and I noted positive and obvious changes in Zeke's speech and understanding. He was now using longer, clearer sentences. He's making a real effort to initiate conversation with us. He has been able to follow instructions given to him for the first time. His fear of dogs is greatly reduced and he has stopped physically lashing out at us. His reading and spelling of key words are next on our agenda with Zeke and we have plans to appoint a tutor one evening per week to assist in helping him to become more able in these areas of communication.

CHAPTER 18:
Zeke's educational achievements up to age 19+

"Just because a man lacks the use of his eyes doesn't mean he lacks vision." Stevie Wonder

At age 16+ Zeke achieved the ASDAN Transition Challenge Certificate.

The certificate reads as follows:

Has successfully completed the Transition Challenge in the following units:

Knowing 'How' – without help; Making Choices-without help; Feeling Good-spoken/signed -without help.

For three years Zeke studied at Haringey Sixth Form College from age 16 to 19. He studied in the Entry and Foundation Department.

At the end of this course he received the Oxford Cambridge and RSA Entry Level 3 (OCR Level 3) qualification

The units he studied involved Life and Living Skills and ICT. These include the following:

Following a simple recipe Shopping for daily living

Recognising time through regular events

Using coins and notes

Participating in a mini-enterprise ICT project at (CONEL)

In 2016 Zeke successfully completed a six-week work placement at Action for Kids community project in Crouch End.

Zeke has also had achievements in out of college activities, for example:

In January 2018 he received the Jack Petchey Outstanding Achiever award through his attendance at Haringey Shed where he studied Dance and Singing.

At the point of graduating from Sixth Form College on June 29, Zeke achieved the OCR Award for Entry Level 3.

At age 19+ Zeke graduated from Haringey Sixth Form College and moved on to New City College in September 2018, where he commenced the 'Pathway towards Independence' course. This course is a progression from Entry Level 3 and its duration is usually two years.

The components in this qualification are as follows:

Completing forms with personal information, Using ICT to produce a text document and using ICT to find information. Functional Mathematics and Functional English, Sports, ICT and Independent Living Skills.

CHAPTER 19:
Photographs of Zeke and his family

"Learning how to get along with other people is vital for our own success and happiness." **John Elder Robinson**

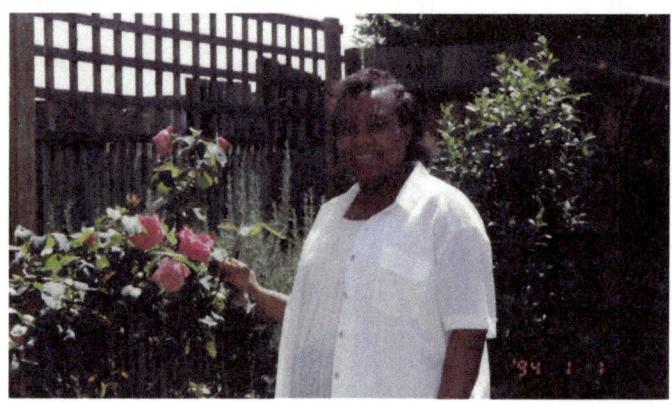

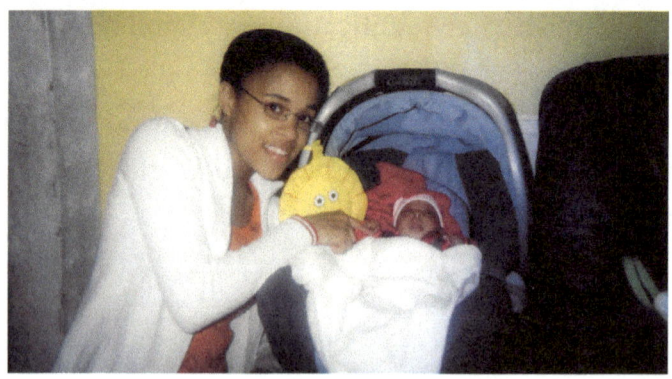

Zeke at six weeks old with his sister

AUTISM – ONE FAMILY'S JOURNEY

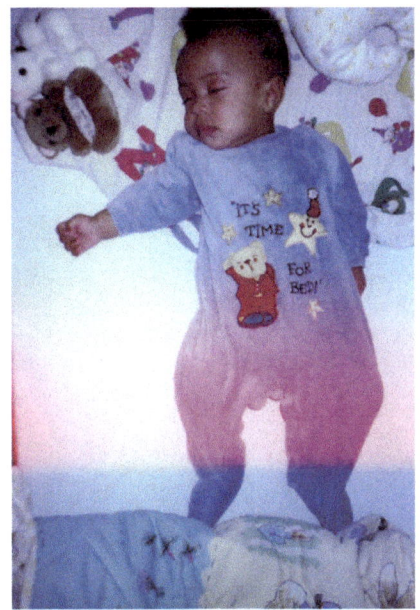

Zeke at 3 months old

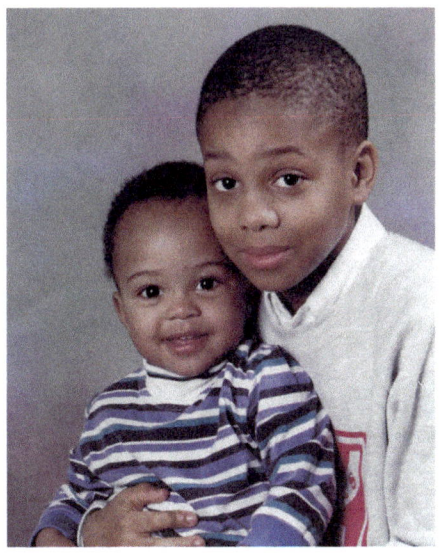

Zeke at 6 months old with his brother

VELORA M. LEVY-SAILSMAN

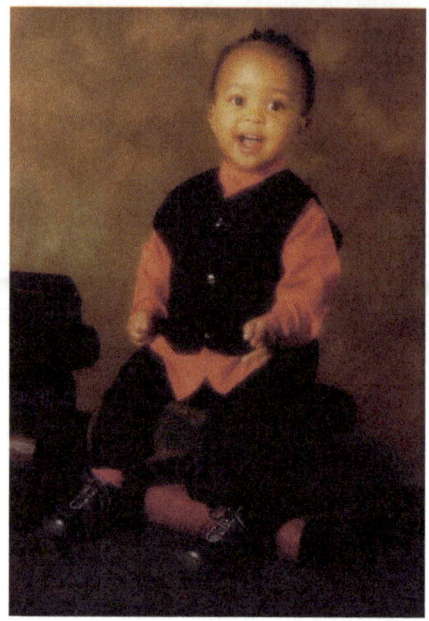

Zeke age 1 year old

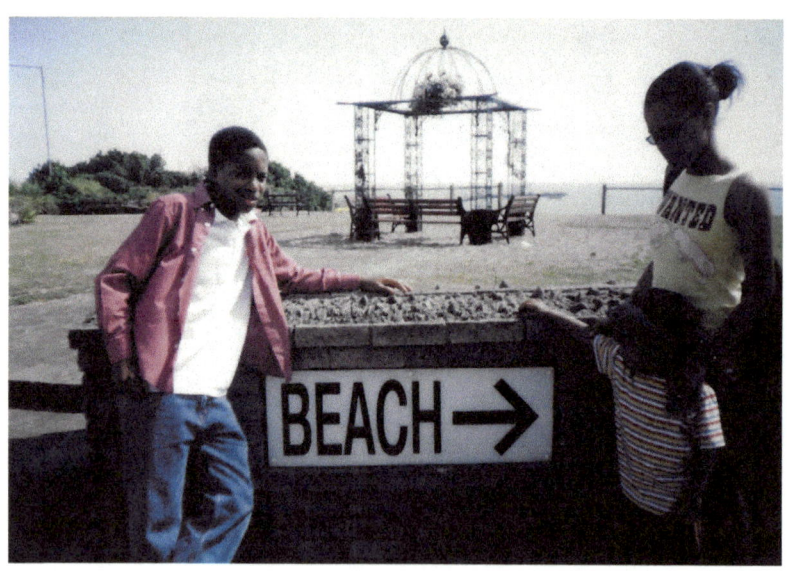

Zeke at age 2 years with his siblings on a day outing in Brighton

AUTISM – ONE FAMILY'S JOURNEY

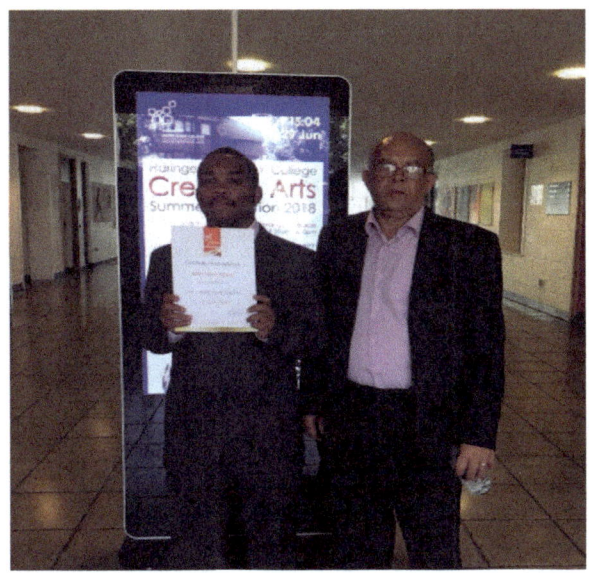

Zeke and his father at his graduation at Haringey 6th Form College

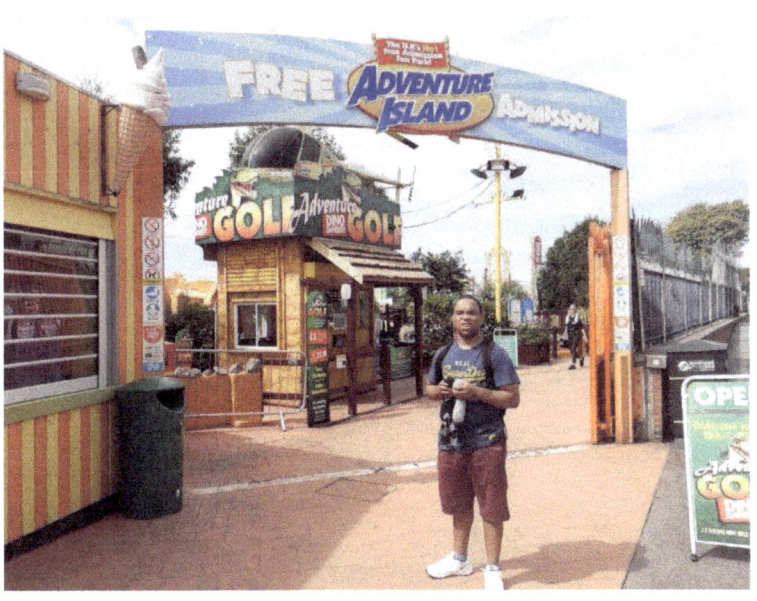

Zeke on a visit to Southend beach with his mother during August 2020

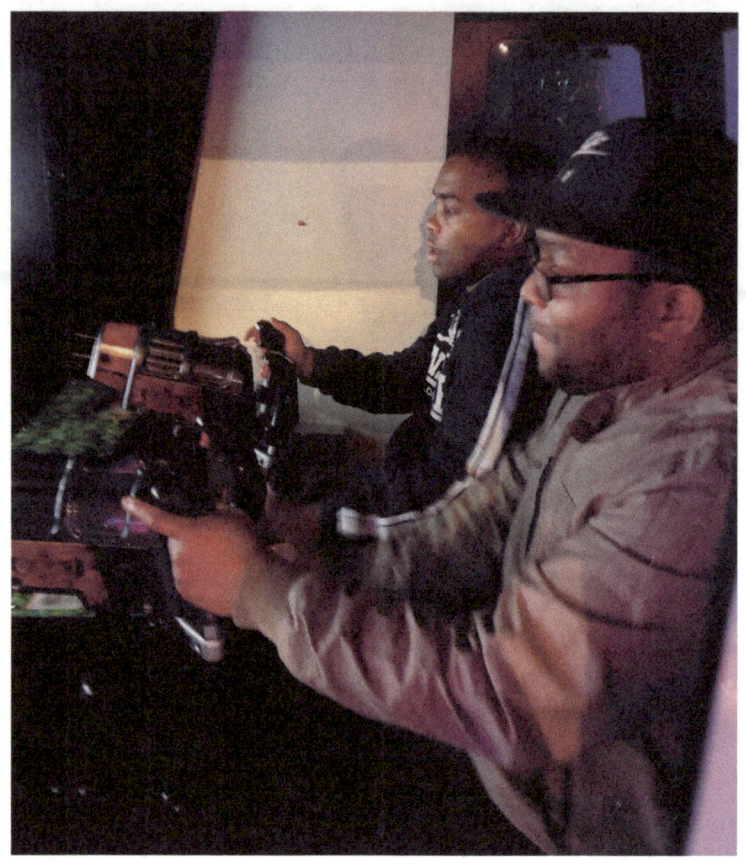

Zeke celebrating his 21st birthday with his brother at Quaser

CHAPTER 20:
Recommendations for paediatric health care workers

"What counts in life is not the mere fact that we have lived. It is what difference we have made to the lives of others that will determine the difference of the life we lead."
Nelson Mandela

Health care workers and paediatric health visitors should ensure that parents and carers understand the importance of making it a priority to encourage face to face talk and mouth awareness from birth with their babies. If the father of the baby is a quiet and non-talkative person it's imperative that babies should not be left solely in his care for long periods of time. Older siblings under 18 years should not be left to care for the baby if the baby is age three years and under. They usually don't have the experience and emotional abilities or intelligence to empathetically care for babies and toddlers.

If Obsessive Compulsive Disorder (OCD) extends to an interest in intimacy the ASD young adult could easily become sexually promiscuous and at times taken advantage of or get exploited by adults much older than themselves. If a young lady should fall for the charm of a man, I suggest that such relationships should be shadowed by a carer showing interest in both parties. The young ASD man should not be trusted with a younger partner than himself because the word 'No' is a word that he will not readily understand.

If the ASD person is also an OCD sufferer (obsessive, compulsive, disorder) who has the tendency to tell lies and, this young adult could be easily believed. In the long term this behaviour could cause confusion and problems for others. These individuals are very deceptive and will be good at covering up unacceptable behaviours such as having a double life without anyone suspecting them. For example they could be happily married with loads of children, holding down a professional job, yet they could be in a long-term homosexual or heterosexual relationship without anyone suspecting or doubting them.

In terms of friendship they will have friends but know how to keep them at arm's length or give the impression to others that they are loyal to their known partner. This type of ASD mother will also encourage her ASD adult son to indulge in extramarital relationships with other women despite having a loving and stable relationship with his wife. Most often these extramarital relationships and the illegitimate children will be kept secret as some ASD adults are very good at concealing the truth and keeping secrets.

CHAPTER 21:
My contribution to young ASD people and their families

'I think a hero is an ordinary individual who finds strength to persevere and endure in spite of overwhelming obstacles.'
Christopher Reeve

First of all, on 4th May 2018 I registered a Community Interest Company (CIC) business at Companies House, under the name of 'Velora Autism Corner' (VAC).

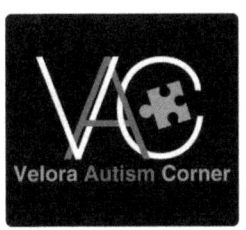

I decided to compile a single leaflet to publicise and market this business. On this leaflet I explained my six provisions which I have in place to assist with the learning and development of youths on the autism spectrum. These provisions will subsequently support the parents or guardians of this target group. However for the benefit of Copy Rights purpose I will only elaborate on one of these programmes in this book.

OUR READING RECOVERY PROGRAMME
I use the following catch phrase 'It's never too late to learn to read' as a means to capture the imagination and attention of parents.
In my publicity leaflet I pose the following question. 'Are you worried that your child has not mastered reading?' Then I reassure them that 'We can help.' I add, 'We will have your child reading at an appropriate level within three months.'

This program will be led initially by a qualified Primary School teacher who is also qualified to teach children with a specific learning difficulty such as autism.

The teacher will meet with the young person and their parent/carer for assessment and observation purposes. It is during this meeting when the registration for the organisation will be completed.

Initially all reading sessions will be held at the home of the young person. A parent or a support worker is expected to be present during each session. The aim is that the teacher's approach will be learnt and practised on a daily basis for 10 minutes, initially by one of the above-mentioned people. When the teacher is ready he or she will request that the young person be accompanied to her office to continue the reading programme there. As each young person becomes more confident in reading they will be encouraged to read in pairs at our weekly youth club.

THE AIMS AND OBJECTIVES OF VELORA AUTISM CORNER READING RECOVERY PROGRAMME

Aims: *The reasons why I've put this programme in place:*
According to recent statistics in the Independent newspaper a large number of youngsters who are diagnosed with autism are leaving secondary schools unable to read. Unfortunately my son Zeke also fit into this category.

The aim of our Reading Recovery Programme is to get youngsters from age 11-25 reading at a reasonable standard or level.

You are no doubt thinking, 'Why not include writing?' Remember, most ASD youngsters are fragmented learners. So I'm sorry to say, in order for them to learn new skills a fragmented or dissected approach should be adapted or put in place.

Having said that, if during these reading sessions the ASD youngster has initiated the interest to do writing, that desire will be gladly encouraged and supported, providing that writing isn't one of their obsessions. However, as the heading of this literature states, the emphasis is 'Reading Recovery'. Whenever possible the youngster will be sensitively re-directed back to his/her reading book.

Fine 'motor skills' development will be practised during our weekly youth club and during our 'Holiday Teen scheme sessions' when all youngsters will get the opportunity to make craft objects based on ideas from various countries.

Objectives: *How the programme will be delivered.*
First of all the teacher will spend some time observing the ASD youngster within his/her home environment, surrounded by their siblings and caregivers. The teacher will talk with family members about specific interests or topic of interest. During these visits the teacher will make detailed written notes of what they are being told by professionals about their ASD youngster.

Most of the interaction between the teacher and the ASD youngster will take place during each reading session. Therefore parents or caregivers should not be concerned if the teacher does not engage much with the youngster before the reading sessions commence.

Step 1:- The teacher will mentally take the ASD youngster right back to the Reception classroom, regardless of their age. The alphabet song must be song. Next the teacher will direct the youngster to the letters on the alphabet board. If this youngster knows all 26 letters of the alphabet the teacher will proceed to establish if he/she knows letter sounds or phonemes.

If this youngster knows these, the next step will be for them to commence reading a book chosen by the teacher but based on a topic that is of interest to that particular youngster.

Step 2: This will involve the youngster reading daily for 30 minutes with his teacher whilst being observed by that chosen family member or support worker, who will be appointed as the person taking over from the teacher and who will be responsible for putting into practice exactly the approach that the teacher has demonstrated in his/her presence on a daily basis, at the same place and time. Please be reminded that, 'a true ASD person cannot tolerate change'.

The teacher, however, will do a weekly follow-up to establish if her learner has learnt certain targeted words which will be based around the first 200 High Frequency Words or frequently used words. Please see below for some of these words. These are in frequency order reading down the columns.

A LIST OF THE FIRST 100 MOST USED WORDS IN THE ENGLISH VOCABULARY

The	That	Not	Look	Put
And	With	Then	Don't	Could
A	All	Were	Come	House
To	We	Go	Will	Old
Said	Can	Little	Into	Too
In	Are	As	Back	By
He	Up	No	From	Day
I	Had	Mum	Children	Made
Of	My	One	Him	Time
It	Her	Them	Mr	I'm
Was	What	Do	Get	If
You	There	Me	Just	Help
They	Out	Down	Now	Mrs

On	This	Dad	Came	Called
She	Have	Big	Oh	Here
Is	Went	When	About	Off
For	Be	It's	Got	Asked
At	Like	See	Their	Saw
His	Some	Looked	People	Make
But	So	Very	Your	An

Step 3:- This will involve the teacher teaching this particular ASD youngster a process in reading called 'phonics and blends'. This process will be introduced like a rhythmic game. For example: 'a b c d e f g h I j k l m n o p q r s t u v w x y z'. Afterwards we will proceed to do the following: 'I say SC; you say…. And the youngster will be expected to repeat the sound for 'SC'.

Step 4:- This will involve this particular youngster continuing to read to his appointed tutor within the home and the teacher giving much attention to sounding out letters in words and recognising the correct word as well as recognising blends.

Step 5:- The goal will be to encourage this particular youngster to continue reading as a habit independently and with a family member.

Step 6:- This goal will be to test the youngster's understanding of the text he's reading by being asked simple questions by his teacher or support worker about the text that has been read.

Step 7:- Marking and assessment of each youngster's reading progress.   When the teacher is satisfied that the youngster has read the chosen paragraph well she will encase that paragraph with a large boxed shape bracket such as [   ] using the same colour ink previously used. The teacher will make a complimentary comment at that bracket as a means to note progress or concerns. Then he or she will put the date and her initials nearby. Finally she will proceed to select the next paragraph that the youngster should proceed to read. Then repeat as above until the whole chapter of that book has been read before moving on to the next chapter.

Further assessment:- A short written comprehension exercise should be prepared by the teacher and given as an independent work for the youngster to complete when each chapter has been read.

Marking of this exercise: - This exercise should be completed by the student within 15 minutes and should be marked by the teacher in the presence of the student. The teacher must <u>explain</u> wrong answers and <u>praise</u> correct answers to them.

The marking system of the reading recovery technique
Extracts taken from Frank Lampard children's books 'Frankies Magic Football as Zeke loves football and is fond of Frank Lampard a famous footballer of the 21st Century.

"Can he swim?" asked the steward, frowning.

"Like a fish," said Frankie.

"All right, then," said the steward. "A few rules. Jackets stay on at *all* times. No standing up in the boats. No splashing with the oars. And no going beyond the buoys." He pointed across the lake to where a line of red inflatables were bobbing in the water.

"Got it," said Frankie.

The steward nodded at the football in Frankie's hand. "Want to leave that with me?"

Frankie clutched the ball tighter. It was falling to bits — the stitching had completely gone down one side.

"I'd better keep it with me, thanks."

"OK, you're good to go," said the steward. He watched Frankie and Kevin climb into the boat with Max. The small craft wobbled under Frankie's feet as he settled on the bench. Louise clambered into a second boat, but Charlie remained on the jetty. He chewed his lip nervously.

"What's the matter?" said Kevin. "Don't tell me you're scared of water!"

"I'm not a great swimmer," said Charlie.

"Don't worry," said Louise,

holding out a hand to him. "You've got a life vest on – and anyway we won't be getting wet."

Charlie stepped into the boat and sat down, smiling weakly.

The steward handed each crew a set of oars. "See you in half an hour," he said, then walked back to his little cabin out of the rain.

Frankie tucked the football under his bench, and saw that Kevin was smirking at him. "Keeping it close, I see," he said.

Frankie ignored him. His brother knew very well what the magic football was capable of, and liked to tease Frankie about it. In fact,

His brother was laughing as he continued to splash the others, but Louise just sank the oars again, and rowed away.

"Great! Let's race!" said Kevin.

With a lot of rocking, he managed to turn the boat around.

"Maybe we should just go back to shore," said Frankie.

Kevin began to thrash the oars as he tried to row. He wasn't very good, but soon they were veering in an uneven course after Louise. Max whined between Frankie's feet.

Kevin looked back over his shoulder, keeping on track. Frankie pulling them in. Max whined and laid a paw across his eyes.

Kevin and Charlie paddled furiously with their hands, scooping up water.

"What's happening?" yelled Kevin, his face twisted with fear.

"It's the magic football!" said Frankie. "Hold on, everyone."

But Kevin must have seen his chance. As the boat's nose dipped into the whirlpool, he jumped clear, grabbing at a branch that was growing over the water. Frankie saw his brother's legs dangling, and then the world lurched over. He tumbled out of the boat.

AUTISM – ONE FAMILY'S JOURNEY

Together, they swam more slowly down into the city. There were fields of limp, dying seaweed covering the seabed, and no fish at all in the water. Complete silence fell over the ruined city.

"Where is everyone?" said Zoe.

At the sound of her voice, a boy with a tail came swimming from under an archway. "Sister!" he cried. "You're back!"

He looked about the same age as Zoe. "Avi! What happened here?" she asked.

"The sharks came," he said sadly. "They took..." He stopped as a huge creaking groan filled the

"So how d'you make it go?" asked Charlie, on his dolphin's back. "Giddy-up, boy!"

The dolphin rolled its eyes. "Actually, you just need to ask politely," the creature told him.

Charlie gasped. "Oh, right. Didn't realise you talked. Er ... go, please?"

"We're very sensitive and clever creatures," the dolphin explained. "Squeeze lightly with your knees. Steer by pressing lightly with your hands. Maybe take off those gloves."

Charlie looked alarmed and Frankie grinned. He nudged his dolphin's flanks and it shot taking part in a football obstacle course – a test of sprinting, dribbling, heading and shooting. He couldn't wait!

As they left the hall through the double doors at the back, Frankie saw the school's Olympic torch burning on its stand in the playground. Mr Donald had told them that the real torch was lit every four years in a place called Olympia in Greece. Runners then carried it in a relay to whichever country was hosting the Games. Sometimes they ran thousands of miles! The torch never went out and symbolized the spirit of the Games.

8

Mr Donald clapped his hands. "Right, parents, please take your places on the sports pitch. Kids – go and get ready. The games will begin in twenty minutes!"

Frankie and his friends warmed up round the side of the school in the shade. They used his magic football, passing it between them, dribbling it around, and heading it back and forth.

"Are you sure it's safe to have your football in school?" said Charlie, stretching to catch it. "You know what it can do." The ball had taken them on adventures all said, opening the car door. "Some time with Mother Nature."

Kevin looked up from his games console. "Yeah, great," he grumbled. "Loads of insects and a lumpy bed."

Frankie unclipped his seat belt, and jumped out of the car. They'd been driving for nearly three hours to reach the holiday camp. Max whined from the back, so Frankie went to let him out too. He sprang out on to the grass.

Frankie breathed in the crisp air of the forest. He couldn't wait to explore the camp. Apparently there were tennis courts, an outdoor heated pool and even a mini theme

4

park. But the best thing about this whole trip was that Louise and Charlie were coming with their families as well.

"Hey, Frankie, give me a hand with the luggage, will you?" asked his dad.

Frankie saw his father struggling with a huge suitcase, and rushed over to help him. Together, they dragged it out of the car. Frankie's football rolled out after it.

"I don't know why you keep that old thing," said his dad. "Didn't we get you a new ball for your last birthday?"

Frankie grinned and picked up

who hobbled forward on a crutch. "You must all stay for a feast," he said. He glared at Kevin. "Even the one who disrespects the Great Spirit."

Frankie's stomach rumbled. He realised he hadn't eaten anything since lunch time, and that seemed a long, long time ago. But they had to get back. Even though the hours here passed differently, their dads were looking for them now. They'd sounded really worried.

"Thank you for the offer," said Frankie, "but we have to leave."

Cywan looked at the floor sadly.

"Will we ever see you again?" he asked.

Frankie didn't want to disappoint him. "I suppose there's a chance we'll come back – one day."

"Don't worry," said Max, placing a paw on Cywan's leg. "The Great Spirit will always be watching over you."

"Oh, please!" said Kevin. "This is ridiculous. Hey, kid." He walked towards Cywan. "Hand over the ball."

But as he tried to kick it from under Cywan's foot, the young boy rolled it back neatly and Kevin fell over on his bum.

disappoint – 123 let down
ridiculous – silly

CHAPTER 22:
Going on holiday with Zeke

'I think a hero is an ordinary individual who finds strength to persevere and endure in spite of overwhelming obstacles.'
Christopher Reeve

Zeke's first holiday was at Euro Disney in Paris. He was ten months old. We travelled by coach from Ponders End to Dover where the coach embarked onto the ferry to Marne-la-Vallée station in Paris Disneyland. Accompanying us were his big sister Kelsey and big brother Cuffie. The one way journey took five hours in total. Zeke slept most of the journey, only waking up to be fed and have his nappy changed. We spent three nights and four days there.

Zeke's second holiday was again in Disneyland Paris when he was twenty-one months old. On this occasion his father Zephie joined us for this trip. This time round, we travelled by the Eurostar train to Marne-la-Vallée station. Firstly we travelled by the underground from Seven Sisters station, changing several times before arriving at Waterloo where we boarded the Eurostar train to Disneyland Paris. Zeke was wide awake for most of this journey which took four hours in total. We spent four nights and five days on this occasion.

Zeke's third holiday was again in Disneyland Paris when he was five years old. On this occasion the only family member absent was big sister Kelsey. Again we travelled by train to Waterloo and from Waterloo to Disneyland Paris. Again Zeke was awake for most of the journey. He did not fuss but sat happily in his buggy facing us.

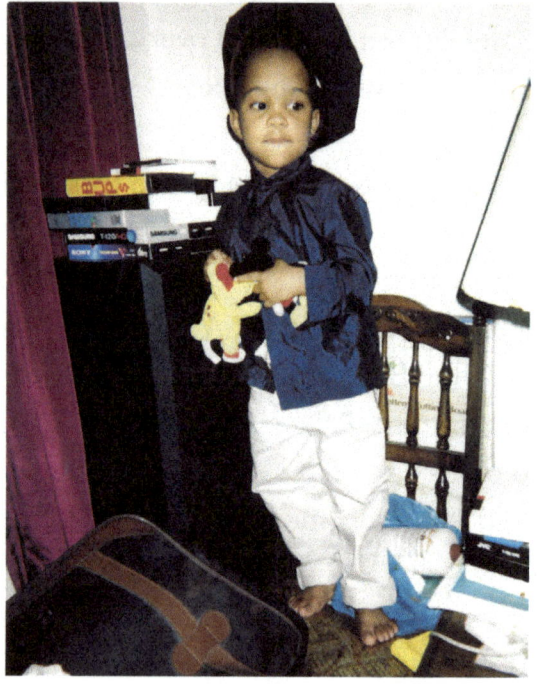

Zeke wearing cousin Donny's taxi cap

Zeke's fourth holiday was again at five years old when he travelled during the month of November by aeroplane for the first time to attend his Godmother Carol's wedding in the

United States of America. Zeke sat beside his older brother Cuffie who was fourteen years old and behaved well. Both lads played computer games and watched movies throughout the flight on our forward and backward journeys. Zeke ate his meals and drank without fussing. We stayed at my cousin Donny and his wife's home for one week and Zeke was the star of the environment.

After the wedding had taken place the four of us went on a bus tour to visit 'Ground Zero'. This is the famous trading centre where the twin towers were deliberately destroyed by aeroplanes plotted by terrorists. Afterwards we went to MacDonald's and had a meal before returning to our cousin's home. Whilst still at cousin Donny's home Zeke initiated wearing Donny's taxi cap and decided to jump up on the bed we had slept on. As he jumped, Donny decided to take pictures of him. Zeke clearly enjoyed himself.

Two days later on our way back to the airport to return to England, Donny drove us to my older sister Nerissa's home in Far Rockaway, which was approximately 30 minutes' drive away. When we arrived at her home the table was laid for us to have a Thanksgiving meal. Zeke was clearly looking forward to sitting down and enjoying the meal but time was against us for boarding our plane on time. I requested to have a packed lunch, which my sister Nerissa prepared for us. After checking in our luggage at the airport, the two lads were happy to indulge in the meal which was made up of turkey and 'hardo' bread. I was happy that Zeke had the opportunity to meet his aunt, her daughter Annie and her grandson Nelson.

At age seven Zeke had his fifth holiday, this time supported by myself and big sister Kelsey. On this occasion we travelled by train to Heathrow then boarded the plane for a nine-hour flight to Jamaica. Zeke was reasonably well-behaved and cooperative. However, he did something that made me question his understanding and awareness of danger.

On noticing the exit sign closest to our aisle on the plane, Zeke spontaneously made a dash for the handle of the door. Luckily I was quick and alert enough to grab him before he could reach the handle of that door. I really felt that Zeke should have known that if the door got opened in mid-air the plane would crash and everyone would perish. I sat him down and talked to him about the danger but I wasn't certain that he understood why I was reprimanding him. Although I was extra vigilant in case he decided to repeat that action, he did not attempt to do so.

Zeke's sixth family holiday was at age nine. This time we opted for a holiday at Alton Towers in the West Midlands, England. On this trip all the family travelled together and Zephie drove us there and drove us back to London three days later. The family consisted of me, dad Zephie, big sister Kelsey and older brother Cuffie.

Zeke's seventh family holiday was at age 12 when he travelled for the third time on an aeroplane again, to Jamaica to attend his big sister Kelsey's wedding to her fiancé Hackhan. This time he was again accompanied by me, his father Zephie and older brother Cuffie.

AUTISM – ONE FAMILY'S JOURNEY

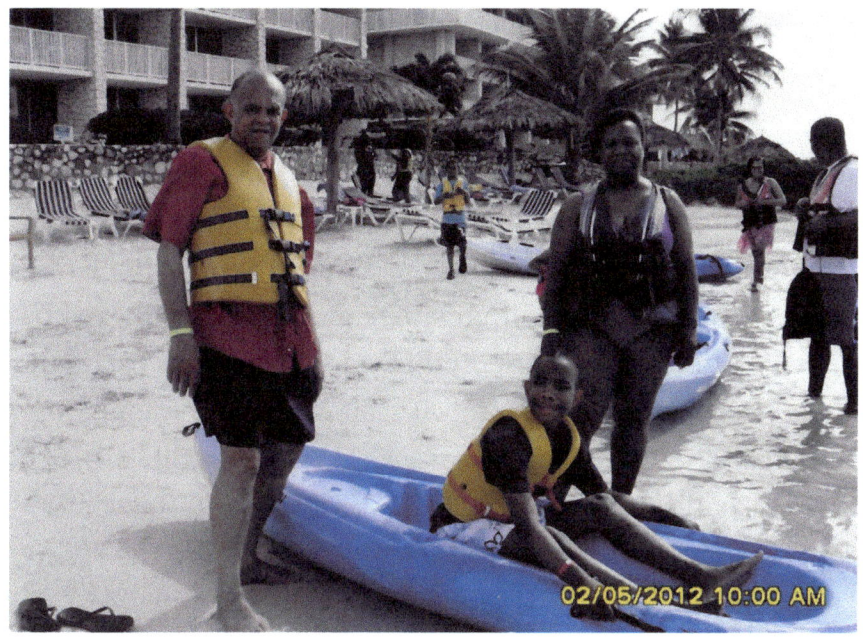

Zeke's eighth family holiday was at age 14 when we travelled by train from Euston to Drayton Manor in the West Midlands. Zeke requested going on the Space Mountain ride on which I accompanied him while his father waited until we returned. I was rather taken aback to see how calm and relaxed Zeke was on the ride. Even when I was terrified and felt as if my stomach was about to pop out of my mouth, Zeke comforted me by saying, 'Mummy don't worry, you be ok,' while holding my arm to comfort and reassure me. When the ride eventually ended and we got off I was feeling dizzy and had to hold on to his father's arm. Zeke was ready straightaway to go on his next ride, which happened to be a miniature train ride around the park looking at various historic scenes.

Zeke's ninth family holiday was at age 19 in August 2018. Zeke visited Euro Disney with me and his father. The four nights and five days' holiday went tremendously well, with Zeke making choices on the rides he wanted to experience and leading us to them. His first ride was the Space Mountain ride but there was an issue with his parents because neither of us wanted to accompany him on that ride. Luckily for us a fault was detected on that ride and it was grounded, undergoing investigation and subsequent repair. We were both pleased, after we had explained to him the problem with his chosen ride, he pointed at another ride, saying, 'that one'. The Flying Saucer seemed a less scary ride so his father Zephie decided to accompany him on that ride while I waited at the side and watched then enjoying the ride.

The next ride Zeke chose was within the Walt Disney studios, which is known as Aladdin's Flying Carpet Ride. Zeke referred to this ride as 'Aladdin'. All three of us went on this ride and we all thoroughly enjoyed it. I was surprised that Zeke did not kick up a fuss or have meltdowns when his father and I suggested at intervals the rides we wanted to experience. Most of the rides involved a minimum of 30 minutes' wait. Zeke waited calmly and patiently until our turn came to go on our chosen ride.

CHAPTER 23:
Situations that caused Zeke to have a meltdown

> *"Everything for me is visual. That's how my head works."* Whoopi Goldberg

In the life of an autistic family a meltdown occurs when the autistic person demonstrates behaviour that is embarrassing to their parents and draws attention to themselves from the public. When Zeke was between 5 and 9 years old he had a habit of screaming out, throwing himself down on the floor and running around the stores and supermarkets when he was told by his parents that he could not have a particular item.

Sometimes this behaviour would be demonstrated if particular items that he was allowed to have were not available in the store or if they had been placed in a different area of the store. We were finding it extremely difficult to tolerate this behaviour so we made the decision that Zeke would no longer accompany anyone to go grocery shopping.

Between the ages of 9 and 12 Zeke would ask repeatedly to be taken shopping to the sports shop. However, we were beginning to find these experiences very disturbing. He would have severe meltdowns if he was told that he couldn't have the whole range of particular football clothing, even if these clothes did not belong to his favourite football team. He simply wanted them and choosing certain ones was not an option for him. He would attempt to grab certain items off the clothes rack and run out of the shop without them being paid for.

Zeke also had meltdowns for other reasons. His father and I had taken him with us on a coach trip to the Isle of Wight with a group of mainly pensioners. It was a holiday of four nights/ five days. But after two nights it was obvious that Zeke had endured enough and quite naturally wanted to return home to London. Zeke was 16 years old when he decided to run away from the resort, which meant we had to chase after him because he was heading for the winding country road. When we caught up with him and attempted to return to the holiday resort he started crying and screaming loudly and obviously drew attention to himself and us. Everyone around came out looking and staring at us, which was extremely embarrassing. When he was physically restrained by his father he started biting and scratching him, leaving obvious bruising to his arms and hands.

That same day when I had decided to give his father a break from him he escaped from my gaze and climbed into a coach that was being boarded by other passengers leaving the resort. He remained standing in the aisle of the coach where the passengers were all seated and the driver was ready to drive off. Luckily the driver was considerate to our feelings and waited fifteen minutes for us to remove him from the coach before driving off. That action only resulted in further loud crying and screaming. This time the wounds were inflicted on me. That day our coach party visited the pier and we all went on a boat ride. He calmed down and enjoyed this experience. Finally the next day was our day for returning to London and Zeke was clearly happy to know this.

SITUATIONS THAT MAKE ZEKE APPEAR QUIRKY
Zeke will throw a ball in the air and spin around twice and catch it before it hits the ground.

At age seven, during Zeke's first holiday in Jamaica, whilst I was busy checking in at the hotel he took the opportunity to run off without me or his sister noticing. His sister was so preoccupied with the issues arising at the reception desk and with our booking arrangements that she did not see him run off. She did not even have a clue about the direction in which he had gone. Once she noticed that he had disappeared she raised the alarm loudly and the staff member who was attending to us said, 'Not to worry, go and look for him and you will be attended to as soon as you return with him.'

This was a frightening experience for me so I said to my daughter, who was twenty-two years old but looked about 16, 'You look around the complex close by, because I don't think he has gone far,' while I looked for the security and welfare officer to report him missing. It took three minutes to walk to this office and I noticed that there was a games arcade in the vicinity. My attention was drawn over there because I knew that Zeke likes to go into places like those. As I entered the small building my eyes met with the supervising staff. She had obviously heard my scream from a distance and was keen to know what was wrong. I instantly told her that my seven-year-old son was missing and I asked her if she had seen a child that age come into the building. She convincingly replied that 'no one so young' had been in there on that day. Then she said, 'You need to report it to security because they are the best persons to assist you in finding him.' Then she pointed out to me a security guard who was standing at the side of the beach looking over in the distance.

I quickly went over to the guard and explained to him, in one breath, that my seven-year-old son has disappeared and I didn't know in which direction he'd gone. He quickly said whilst pointing, 'Look over there, is that him?' Instantly I recognised my son, although by now he was wearing just his briefs and was dancing to the reggae music that was being played.

Standing about two metres away from him was his sister, who was just standing by holding his clothes and trainers in her hands, watching him with a smile on her face. I was so happy that he had been found so quickly and that he was well. I quickly went over to where my daughter was standing and said loudly for him to hear, 'Free at last, Zeke!?' I next asked his sister where she had found his belongings. She explained that he had left a trail from where he had disappeared, so she simply picked up each item of clothing until she came to the last item, where she saw him on the beach in the sand, dancing to music.

My thoughts reflected on the children's story called *Hansel and Gretel* who left pieces of bread as a trail to lead them back to where they had come from. When the music had stopped, we both went over to Zeke and we both let him know how disappointed we were with him for running off. In other words, I told him off for running away without asking permission to go, but Zeke did not utter a word. He stretched out his hand and reached for his clothes, one by one, and put them on except his trainers. I happily held him by the hand and tried to explain how scared and frightened he had made us feel and told him not to run off like that again. We all went back to the hotel reception desk and, as the staff had promised, our registration was quickly completed and we and our luggage were escorted to our hotel accommodation.

Another quirky way Zeke has is that he likes the idea of being in control of certain things around the home. For example, he likes to control the television remote control and choose the television programmes that anyone sitting in the lounge should watch, even though he will be upstairs playing on his choice of technology equipment such as iPad, phone and laptop. Despite our discreteness in changing the television channel while he is upstairs, Zeke will know and he will quickly rush downstairs and switch the television back to the channel he had previously chosen for everyone in the room to watch. Upon placing the remote control at the place where he had put it previously he will assert his authority by looking everyone straight in the eye and saying, 'Leave it!'

Another quirky way that he has is a habit of waking up very early in the mornings, at 4am, taking a bath or shower then getting dressed and going back to bed and sleep until 6am. He will then have a bowl of cereal and a cup of mint tea for his breakfast, all prepared by himself.

ZEKE'S LOVE FOR JESUS AND FOR THE CHURCH

Zeke has a genuine love for Jesus and for the church. Since the age of 12 he has been showing tremendous interest in attending our local Apostolic church and listening to the preaching and participating appropriately in singing and quizzes.

At home he is usually the first member of the family to get ready for Sunday service. He knows when the morning service starts and makes sure he's never late arriving at church. There's been a couple of times when he knew he would be late for church because of us. On these occasions he left home in a hurry and when we eventually arrived at the church ten minutes later, he was seen sitting comfortably beside members of the church with whom we would usually sit. From as early as age 12 he would comment to us that people made Jesus sick. When I shared this dialogue with the pastor of our church, he looked at Zeke and added, 'They murdered him.' Recently Zeke has reminded me to pray. He has a short personal prayer which he repeats most nights before going to bed.

At home he likes to have the Christian channel *Premier Radio* playing in the background whilst he's engaged with other activities. He will purposely leave this programme playing when he's leaving the house to go to college and other places, particularly when he knows someone will be at home for the day. After 10.30pm every Saturday he ensures that no other programme is being played on the television other than a Christian channel where scripture reading and teaching is being given. On Sundays he's first to go downstairs. He will then put this same channel on from as early as 6 am. When we eventually go downstairs we will then be met with the singing of Christian songs as well as bible reading and teaching.

It's comforting to me to know that Zeke has some knowledge of who God is. I now regard it my duty to work with him to build onto the knowledge that he already has about our God, Jesus the Saviour of the world. I strongly believe that if he knows who God is, should his father and I say farewell to the world before he does, he knows that God will take good care of him and he will know the power in prayers to God.

In 2004 J Smith and W McSherry write in the Journal of Advanced Nursing about *Spirituality and Child Development: a concept analysis* (available in the Wiley Online Library). These writers are healthcare professionals who have worked with children.

They are familiar with the work of child development theorists such as Piaget (1952) who wrote about the stages of cognitive development and Erik Erikson (1963). Erikson has been described as an 'ego' psychologist who is regarded as developing one of the most popular and influential theories of development, although it is said that his theory is impacted by Sigmund Freud, the respected psychoanalyst. The main difference between these two theorists is that Erikson's theory focuses on psychosocial development and Freud's is centred on psychosexual development.

Smith and McSherry have both argued that if children are to be given the opportunity to develop their full potential, it's important that they are exposed to spiritual beliefs and practices.

In reference to my son Zeke, he appears to have had a wealth of grounding in the Christian faith beliefs and practices. He regularly participates in the Lord's Supper, listens to the various teachings in the bible around the ten commandments, fruits of the spirit, baptism, fasting, testimony and the importance of prayer. Zeke also has his favourite praise and worship songs.

CHAPTER 24:
Medical negligence claim

"Do the best you can and never stop" Steven Wiltshire

The perusal of a medical negligence claim is an idea I have given much thought about over a number of years. Personally, since the age of 22 I received excellent care from the NHS so I didn't want to act in ways that would appear to be ungrateful. However, I want parents of young children, particularly parents of children with additional needs, to make a stand for them. At the back of my mind I believe that my son's ear, nose and throat (ENT) medical needs were neglected by a specific medical team and I <u>strongly believe that</u> they should be held accountable for their failings.

On the part of the above team of medics, Zeke's medical needs in my opinion were neglected because they appear to believe that he had autism, as an additional learning needs. Once I was confident that the above was my belief, I had no further option but to pursue a medical negligence claim. I took this action, simply to raise awareness of what sometimes happen to certain children who appear to have learning difficulties.

In this chapter my arguments are based on The Report of the Liability claim, Breach of Duty and Causation to the care my son Zeke received from the assigned Paediatrician and Ear Nose and Throat consultant.

When an expert witness was asked to comment on the outcome of my son Zeke undergoing an MRI upper body scan earlier than he did, given the ongoing concerns about his hearing expressed by his mother and the fact that grommets had been suggested by an independent ENT specialist as early as 2001, the following was her response.

'An upper body scan earlier than 14.1.2005 would have picked up persistent paranasal sinus mucosal disease. She added that, the most likely contributory cause of this problem at this young age is recurrent adenoiditis, caused by upper respiratory tract infections. The expert witness further added that, the MRI scan, could have led to an earlier surgical intervention which would involve Zeke having adenotonsillectomy and grommet insertion.'

When this same expert witness was asked the following question:

'Do you consider that Dr B. breached her duty of care in June 2005 by failing to report to the family that Zeke's upper body scan in January 2005 indicated that he had paranasal sinus mucosal disease?'

The following was her response: 'Yes, I consider that Dr B. had breached her duty of care. The relevance of paranasal mucosal disease of the sinuses was not appreciated by Dr B.

and this resulted in an almost two-year delay before Zeke underwent definitive surgery of Adenotonsillectomy, removal of adenoids and tonsils. Grommet insertion was also placed in the eustachian tubes of his ears.'

Question 3 asked the following: 'If so, what action should Dr B. have taken, as a minimum, in order to comply with her duty of care to Zeke?'

The expert witness replied: 'Had Dr B. realised the relevance of persistent paranasal sinus disease, she would have referred Zeke to an ENT surgeon who, given the history of recurrent upper respiratory tract infections and speech delay as a result of recurrent intermittent glue ear, would have recommended adenotonsillectomy and grommet insertion.'

In question 4 the expert witness was asked: 'If, in June 2005, Dr B. had reported the MRI scan fully, both to the family and to the family's GP:

a) What treatment would Zeke have undergone?' The expert witness' response was as follows: 'The most likely intervention would have been a referral back to the ENT surgeon for further reassessment and consideration of surgical intervention in terms of adenotonsillectomy and grommet insertion.' When she was asked the following: b) 'How soon would he have undergone the treatment?' The following was her response: 'Considering the longstanding nature of the problem, he would have undergone the treatment sooner than 2007, most likely in 2005.'

In question 5 she was asked the following: 'Do you have any concerns over the standard of the performance of the adenotonsillectomy and grommet insertion procedure?' The expert witness' response was as follows: 'No, the procedure was performed to a competent standard.'

In question 6 she was asked the following: 'Do you have any other concerns about any of the care afforded to Zeke?' The expert witness' answer was as follows: 'The delay in the diagnosis of recurrent glue ear and hearing loss as a result of frequent upper respiratory tract infections meant that Zeke's diagnosis of autism and its subsequent treatment with Concerta was delayed. The delay also most likely affected his language development and impacted on his cognitive skills.'

In question 7 the expert witness was asked the following: 'Bearing in mind the medical and schooling report of Zeke's improved behaviour following his eventual grommet insertion, how might his development have improved if he had undergone this procedure at the time identified in your answer to question 4(b)?' The expert witness' answer to this question was as follows: 'Zeke would have improved because he would have had an earlier diagnosis of Autistic Spectrum Disorder. It appears that it was not entirely clear whether the diagnosis of autism was a separate diagnosis or secondary to his past hearing loss. This has been alluded to or mentioned casually by Dr L. The evidence, however, suggests that autism is a separate diagnosis and that hearing loss does not cause autism. However, delay in the diagnosis of hearing loss can, and failure to treat it promptly can, delay the diagnosis of autism which means that the child's treatment for autism is also delayed.' For me Dr. L's opinion was that my son had autism therefore there was no need to investigate a possible ENT problem.

These answers above by the expert witness confirm in my mind that the delay in treating my son for his hearing loss resulted in my son developing speech delay early in his development. In my opinion, this same failure to treat the infection in his nasal cavity would have caused excruciating pain which would manifest itself as hyperactivity and the inability to sit and concentrate. Coupled with not being able to hear what people around him were saying would have affected his cognitive and thinking skills. These symptoms are common signs of autism. Therefore in my mind's eye, failure to treat Zeke's adenoids, tonsils and he having recurrent ear infections over a considerable amount of years increased the severity of autism in my son.

Finally, in question 8 the expert witness was asked the following: 'What other benefits would Zeke have enjoyed if he had undergone the adenotonsillectomy/grommet insertion procedure earlier?'
The following were the expert witness' answers:
1. Zeke would have experienced less pain and suffering from his recurrent ear infections.
2. The diagnosis of autism would have been made earlier.
3. Concerta medication would have commenced earlier.
4. Zeke would have received targeted learning at the nursery.

5. His school would have been better informed so that appropriate measures could have been put in place to address Zeke's behavioural and learning difficulties.

In summary:

" I'm where I am because I believe in all possibilities"
Whoopi Goldberg

I've given a definition of autism and have listed historically the different types of autism. I have attempted to include theories about the origin and symptoms of autism. I've also attempted to include theories presented by Cognitive Psychologists such as Sigmund Freud, Jean Piaget, Vygotsky and Bowlby. I've described the symptoms of autism and the processes involved in diagnosing the condition. I've explained the difference between Asperger's syndrome and autism. I've stressed the importance of early diagnoses and intervention in regards to ASD. I've highlighted that a larger percentage of African and Caribbean boys are diagnosed as being autistic than boys from other cultures or races in the United Kingdom.

I've also highlighted that a particular outer London borough is renowned for having a larger amount of children being diagnosed with autism in comparison to other London boroughs. I've described the attempts being made by particular organisations in the island of Jamaica to eradicate the taboo and stigma surrounding autism.

I've outlined my journey in great detail from pregnancy to raising my son who has ASD/ADHD to the age of 19. I've attempted to give reassurance that autism is not anyone's fault and that it is a genetic issue as well as possibly other factors which contribute to the ASD syndrome. I've attempted to encourage families to embrace their ASD child and regard them as a beautiful gift. In my conclusion you will read about my personal opinion in regards to what I think is the cause of my son's autism.

I also attempted to explain why I know that I did not fit the description of 'a freezer or refrigerator mum' towards my baby. A 'freezer mum' is a mother who is not emotionally attached to her baby or toddler. She does not naturally cuddle or kiss her baby. She's also not noticeably emotional to her baby. She mainly takes care of the baby's physical needs such as feeding, changing nappies and putting the baby to sleep. She doesn't appear concerned for the child if the baby is crying or appears to be unsettled. She's rarely seen playing or talking with her baby. She also doesn't value the importance of rocking her baby or tapping the back of the baby to burp the baby or for putting the baby to sleep.

CONCLUSION:

"There are enough people in the world who are going to write you off. You don't need to do that to yourself."
Susan Boyle

Regardless of all the arguments and facts I have presented in the earlier parts of this book, I strongly believe that my son's symptoms of autism developed as a result of severe hearing loss during his early years. This hearing loss developed as a result of evidential mistakes not being identified by the hospital paediatricians and Ear Nose and Throat Specialist, until the age of six years.

I had concerns that my son was having problems with his ears from as young as six months old. One particular ENT specialist discharged Zeke from her clinic on four consecutive occasions without even bothering to examine his ears. At first I believed Zeke was experiencing severe pains because he was crying frequently in his sleep.

My first appointment to the family's GP resulted in being told that the possible reason for him crying in his sleep could be because he was having bad dreams. Our visits to the GP were becoming unusually frequent so she decided to perform a thorough examination on him. This process included ears, nose and throat, chest, heart, pulse and reflexes. As a precaution he was referred to the Paediatrics team at our named hospital; the hospital in which he was born.

Whilst remaining under the care of this hospital he was referred to our local Primary Care Trust clinic. Routine hearing tests were done but all concluded that he had sufficient hearing for normal speech to develop. I was never satisfied with the decision or conclusion of the ENT specialist because my son was not responding to his name being called when he was not facing the caller.

In addition he was not following instructions as well as his two older siblings were able to do when they were his age at ten months onwards. Despite my suspicion that he had a hearing impairment, he was able to say some single words such as mum, dad, sister, baba, hello, thank you, hot, cold, bottle, cup, spoon, water and a few more single words. He could also initiate as well as imitate and say two-word sentences such as daddy come, daddy gone, I eat, I drink, and a few more.

However, a drastic change occurred in my son's speech shortly after he was given the triple jab of the three-in-one MMR vaccination. The change was instantly noticeable to me, his father his older sister and brother. Within forty-eight hours of receiving that vaccination, he had stopped saying two-word sentences and was only saying a reduced number of single words, which further reduced and regressed to babbling. It was decided by the GP that he should be examined by a private ENT specialist called Mr H who, after completing a series of tests, explained that our son was experiencing fluctuating hearing loss. This was due to recurrent ear and throat infections. Mr H also found that his left ear was his good ear.

I have maintained and will continue to argue that there are two contributing factors to my son developing autism. One: he already had a combination of infections in his systems. As a result of these ENT infections he was being prevented from hearing words clearly. Two: the three-in-one MMR vaccinations, combined with the ENT infections already in his body, would have been too much for his body's psychological state and immune system to cope with. Hence he began to display symptoms of autism - regressed speech and hyperactive behaviour issues.

When comparing the standard of education for ASD students within our home borough in England with that of Jamaican mainstream schools, Jamaica's schools are better at meeting the educational needs of ASD children. Within schools in our home borough ASD children are given a poor deal. Senior management and teachers are quick to suspend and expel ASD children, particularly boys from African Caribbean origin, from their mainstream school due to disruptive behaviour.

In England the teachers make every effort to have ASD children transferred to specialist provisions. Within Jamaica's mainstream school every effort is made by senior management, class teachers and other staff to meet the educational and behavioural needs of ASD children within mainstream schools. In Jamaica, the decision to have an ASD child transferred to a specialist school or other provision is therefore only made if the child is experiencing bullying and if parents have expressed a preference for a specialist provision.

However, in terms of knowledge of ASD, the ordinary or uneducated British public have a greater awareness of this condition than the Jamaican 'lay' and uneducated public. As a result the British general public are more empathic towards subjects with this condition than are the Jamaican uneducated general public. Therefore it's greatly desired that more drastic measures are put in place to educate the general Jamaican public about ASD so that they will become more accepting and empathetic to the needs and symptoms of people with ASD, their parents and carers.

Perhaps this training could commence with extended families of persons with ASD who will hopefully be equipped to impart their new knowledge to neighbours, friends, church members, work colleagues and associates in other social circles. Volunteers could be encouraged to work in special schools.

Already within Jamaica, all special schools have been linked to a mainstream school whereby a selected group of children with ASD join a mainstream class for lessons one day per week. I recommend that vice-versa, a selected group of mainstream children could have lessons in a special school alongside children with ASD. Special arrangements could also be made for children with ASD to attend churches with support as well as other appropriate community initiatives. I found the latter to be effective for my son's learning and development in England.

As part of the training and education of candidates with ASD they should be taken shopping to large supermarkets and market stalls so that vendors are aware of their existence and indirectly learn more about their needs, abilities and existence. Under no circumstances should they be hidden away from the public, as was historically done, when taboo and stigma were acceptable for the majority of people.

Being visible to the public is both beneficial to persons with ASD as well as to the general public. Persons with ASD also need to learn about the personality of non-ASD or neurotypical subjects. Persons with ASD will learn social skills by observing how the general public deals with difficult and unpleasant situations.

Throughout all societies, people with ASD should be supported at all times because certain types of people with criminal intent will take the opportunity to abuse and exploit them, if they are seen to be unsupported when out and about in the environment. Persons with ASD are vulnerable because they don't usually have the level of social and mental capacity, understanding or spirit of discernment to know when someone has criminal tendencies or plans to inflict harm, exploit them or to take advantage of them.

Finally, wide-scale research needs to be carried out within all schools, particularly those in my home borough which is an outer London borough. My specific borough needs to clarify two issues that are of concern to me.

One: Why are so many children in my home borough getting diagnosed with autism in comparison to other London borough schools?

Two: Additional research needs to be done in the schools in this same borough to establish the reason why a greater number of African and Caribbean black boys are being diagnosed with ASD than their counterparts from other cultures.

' I ASK MYSELF THIS QUESTION, 'WAS I A FREEZER OR REFRIGERATOR MUM?'

I have done a thorough soul and self-searching in regards to whether I did not interact well with my son Zeke effectively when he was a baby. I can confidently say I was in fact the mum who could have been an 'over the top' mum. Since the day I gave birth to Zeke I would hold him in my arms giving him cuddles, kisses and talks to him whilst looking him in the eyes, stroking his cheeks, forehead, whole head, ears, arms, fingers, toes and feet.

If he seemed to have a full tummy I would stroke his tummy. After feeding him I would stroke and pat his upper, middle and lower back. to help him to burp. If he seemed to be constipated I would also stroke and pat his lower back as a means to give him comfort and assistance to free himself.

I would talk to him in a girlish and playful way where I would capture smiles and sounds from him. That made me feel happy when he responded to my interactions. He was a happy, cooing and smiley baby who made lots of cooing sounds and reacted with his whole body and smiles as I or other family members played with him. I encouraged the immediate family to do the same with him, especially when I had to leave to prepare meals or complete other chores around the home.

His sister Kelsey and older brother Cuffie were excited to have a younger baby brother, so playing with him was continuous and exciting for baby Zeke. His father was the calmer and quieter one of the family, but he would happily sit with Zeke in his arms and speak with him and at times watch certain children's programmes on television with him.

Are people from the African race more embarrassed to have an ASD child in their families? Do they maintain a greater taboo and stigma about ASD children in their families than do other races?

In my opinion these conversations need to be had at local level and at national level to educate all cultures in England with a well-resourced social services sector, where families with such children are supported financially.

Families that have children or adults with ASD are encouraged to employ support workers to support them in the community by taking them out into public places to access many learning facilities and opportunities. As a result parents and other family members are encouraged to follow suit, especially if the people with ASD are requesting or making attempts to visit these places independently.

However, in poor countries where social services are limited, children and adults with ASD are more likely to remain at home and not be taken out to experience public provisions and interactions. In addition, families are less likely to speak about their ASD children with people outside of their homes because they do not seem to be excelling in anything worth speaking about.

Based on the isolated case involving my son Zeke, I'm confident to say that the hospital paediatrician who was assigned to his care 'mucked up' because it appears that he deliberately gave us the incomplete result of the MRI scan and then discharged our son from his clinic. Luckily I was prepared to request a second opinion on the initial scan reading of my child one year later.

If necessary I would have sought the involvement of a private external radiographer and paediatrician whose appointment would be to review the MRI scan reading.

What is greatly needed for parents and guardians of people with ASD, be they young children or adults, are 24/7 support departments and sites or 'drop-in' centres with qualified staff and experienced volunteers. Situations have arisen at the weekends or at nights whereby my son Zeke became unmanageable, for example screaming, shouting, crying and breaking things for no obvious reason.

In these instances he would break the glass in doors and windows at home, which at times resulted in him cutting himself. During these episodes of 'meltdown' his father and I became scared, frightened and confused because we didn't know where to go for help.

If there were off-duty social workers 'on call', they were only available to speak on the phone and take a verbal report from us, the parents, while Zeke would be ranting and physically attacking us in the background.

If the above-mentioned provisions were in place then youths with similar conditions and issues as Zeke could have been brought there. The parents are then given some breathing space or respite, while the professionals attempt to establish the actual reasons why there has been a sudden change in his behaviour. We were left to deal with difficult situations on our own. When I sought assistance from staff at Zeke's secondary school or made complaints about the lack of support, I was usually confronted with ridicule, snobbery and made to feel that I was the problem and not our child with ASD.

I also strongly believe it should be made easier for parents to transfer their children from their home borough school to another borough , particularly if they believe that their children aren't making sufficient progress in that school or if previously planned Individual Education Plans (IEP) aren't being adhered to. When children are transferred to another school or college all requirements as stated in the Education

Health Care Plan should be easily transferred to the child's new educational establishment. For example, the home borough should put transport and speech and language therapy requirements in place.

The receiving borough educational establishment should also not discriminate against these migrating students by depriving them from having speech and language therapy as well as formal 'travel training'. In the meantime the receiving educational establishment should have a strategy in place to make sure that the child's home borough produces the funding without delay.

I believe that technology is a contributing factor to ASD, especially in boys. The child with ASD has a tendency to zoom into their own world in the same way they zoom into the computer whilst detaching themselves from the people or activities around them. I also strongly believe that the type of autism that my son and many more children have developed is due to a lack of early medical intervention.

Let me elaborate further. The brain is like a sponge in many ways. In the same way that a young healthy human brain absorbs knowledge and information, so it is, when there is infection in the system. Particularly, when an infant has an ear, nose and throat infection.

In my opinion, when the infection in areas such as these are left untreated by the appropriate and effective medical intervention and medicine, what happens is this: the infection travels up to the brain and begins to destroy the cells in the brain. It depends which areas of the brain it occupies and festers to cause damage. All humans have these areas in their brain. The frontal lobe, which is the forehead area, the parietal area which is located at the back of the head, the occipital area which is located in the middle of the skull , the left side of the brain which is responsible for speech development and the right side of the brain enables creativity development.

Let's visualise the tonsils, at the back of the neck, becoming infected and remaining untreated by an effective medicine. The tonsils will become swollen and enlarged and obviously very painful. The lungs will also become infected. Gradually this infection begins to move upwards towards the brain. Firstly it will infect the nasal cavity, here the adenoids will become diseased. The inner ear canals will also become diseased.

Finally it will infect the various lobes of the brain. When this infection reaches the left side of the brain, instantly it begins to cause damage to the speech and memory centres. Victims of these unpleasant circumstances, such as young babies, will be in severe pain. But unfortunately, because they have not yet developed speech, they will not be able to tell anyone that they are feeling pain. They will become irritable and cry a lot even when they're asleep. They may often be off their food but may tolerate having drinks. These were the experiences of our son Zeke. Lastly, its important to note that Zeke is the first in his family lineage to have experienced speech difficulties and limited cognitive skills. This knowledge has led me to conclude that the main contributing factor to Zeke's autism is fluctuating hearing loss due to ongoing untreated ear nose and throat infections coupled with nodules on his voice box.

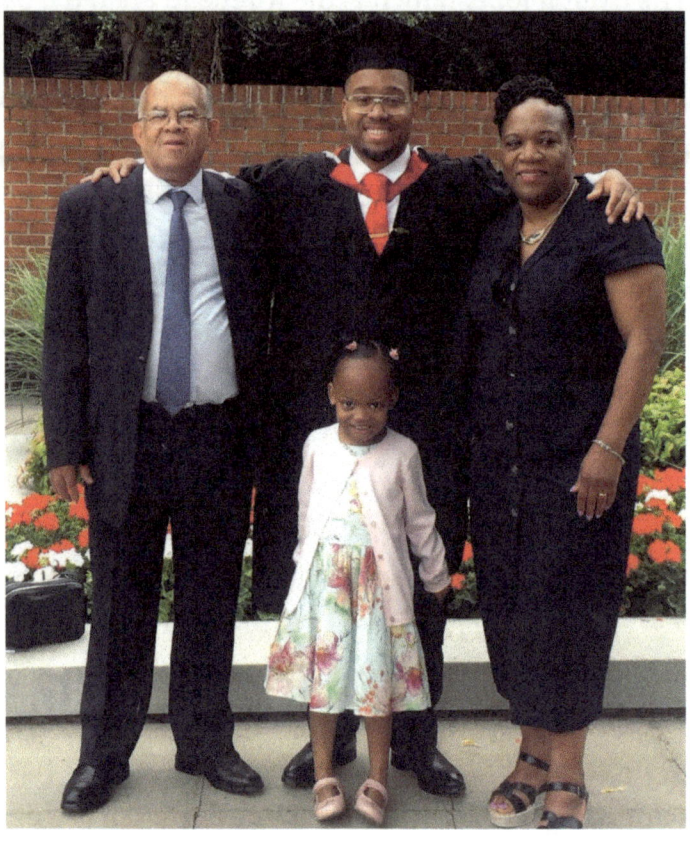

Zeke's parents and niece attending his older brother Cuffie's graduation in July 2019

Glossary of abbreviated words, unusual words and their meanings, explanations etc.

1. ADHD - Attention Deficit Hyperactivity Disorder
2. Pervasive dysfunction - A term used when the medics are unsure if the presented condition in the child might eventually lead to a diagnosis of autism
3. Concerta - Medication that reduces hyperactive behaviour
4. ASD - Autistic Syndrome Disorder
5. OCD – Obsessive Compulsive Disorder
6. Tourette's syndrome - The use of inappropriate language
7. Dyspraxia - Clumsiness
8. Fragile X - An inherited condition which presents learning difficulties
9. A freezer or refrigerator mum - A mum who does not cuddle and play with her new born babies
10. Scaphocephaly -The early merging of the skull in babies
11. Mucosal disease - Disease of the adenoids of the nasal cavities in babies and young children.

VELORA M. LEVY-SAILSMAN

REFERENCES/RESOURCES

- Autism Chronicle 2008/2014 -Mia Chung
- Windsor School of Special Education, Jamaica, April 2017
- Pathways through Autism, Jamaica, April 2017
- Sure Foundation Education Centre, Jamaica, April 2017
- Education Ministry tackles autism, Jamaica Observer .com July, 2017
- The Guardian July 2017 - Article: What my son's autism has taught me. By David Mitchell
- www.webmd.com/brain/autism/development-disorder April 2017
- Completed questionnaires by parents with ASD children Aug 2017
- www.Ted.com
- ASD advocated video talk: Temple Grandin; Rosie King – How Autism freed me from myself.
- www.watchmojo.com
- www.veloraautismcorner.com

Follow me on social media: Facebook=velora levy; velora autism corner, Instagram, Twitter, LinkedIn and www.veloraautismcorner.com

Facebook and Instagram: Velora Autism Corner and Velora Levy

Author of the book: 'She caused the lightning to strike': published 2016 by Create Space and available for purchase at amazon.com

AUTISM – ONE FAMILY'S JOURNEY

This book is also available as an audio and in Kindle format.
Business Email: manager@veloraautismcorner.com
Founder and CEO of Velora Autism Corner CIC foundation

COVID PANDEMIC ANTHOLOGY STORIES

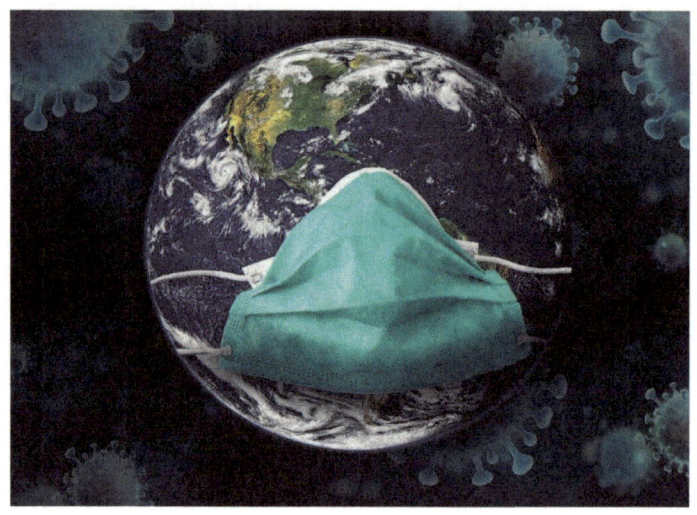

By Six Members of Velora Autism Corner C.I.C

"To be successful, you have to be out there, you have to hit the ground running." Sir Richard Branson

Contents

Something radical was changing in my body By Nathaniel Charles	251
I'm autistic and covid has closed my favourite places Zeke's frequently used Covid-19 words By Zeke Sailsman	258
The spread of covid-19 around the world By Kenneth Osei-tutu	261
My Covid Life By Herald Essuman	264
Safe through the storm By Valerie Ekoli and Kael	267
The Corona virus and Miraculous me By Velora M. Levy-Sailsman	270

VELORA M. LEVY-SAILSMAN

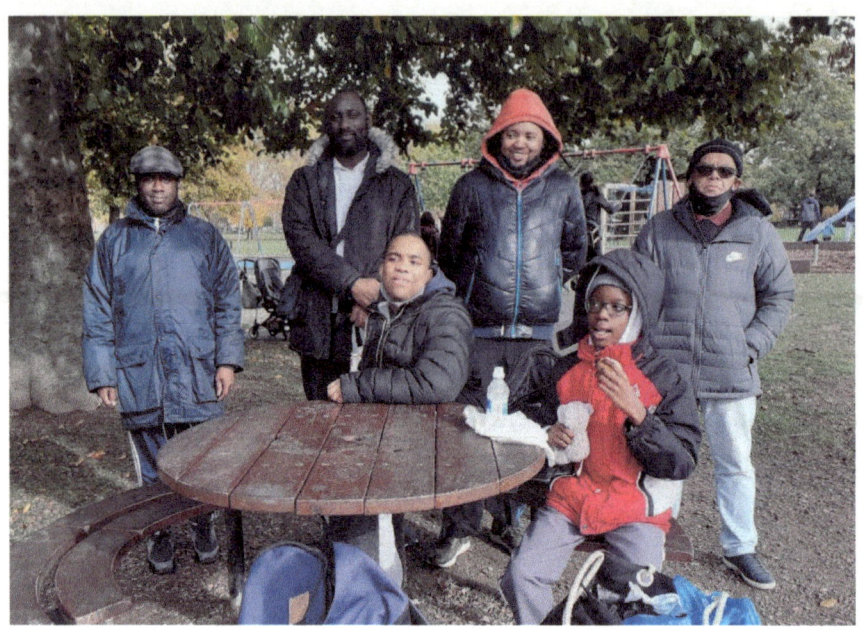

First from the left is Herald, second is Zeke sitting beside Kael and Nathaniel standing between them

SOMETHING RADICAL WAS CHANGING IN MY BODY

By Nathaniel Charles

Thursday 19 March 2020 was known as a glooming chilly day when the atmosphere felt like a spiral attack. It was an adventurous day for a vulnerable passenger that can have a low immune system, who was travelling to the other side of London for work in Ponders End. When he reached his destination to the family home for whom he works, there was the news that he was in a terrible meltdown due to the outbreak that was happening across the UK borders.

His manager looked at him in disbelief as she was worried about everyone's safety as her husband was coming from the outskirts of London where he works. She already had plans to go out to conduct some work-related issues. She had warned me and her excited as well as hulk of anxious son to stay indoors and have fun, until she returns from this chilly, cloudy doomsday weather.

An hour and a half into work, I started to feel a cold sensation in my body which didn't feel right at all. Even though, I was having a non-productive day with the young man. In typical fashion I carried on with a fighting spirit to entertain my client who I'm helping to develop his social skills in various ways. As it came closer to lunch time we decided to have a delicious and delightful meal. As it came to relax mode to digest his system, I decided to rest my body on the long, puffed-up couch that can be a little uncomfortable at times.

But as I was lying down, my body decided to turn cold and I felt like a shivering newborn animal being born into a new world. My symptoms became clear that something radical was changing within my body. Things became uneasy and edgy later on and when my boss returned from the cold and chilly atmosphere, she was still worried about everyone that she cares for. Then thirty minutes later her lovely well-mannered husband walked through the door.

The pandemic started to creep into our minds where we all had a brief discussion on how we should continue to support one another for the next day. So around 3pm local time we thought it was best for business that they sent me home. The government of Mr Boris Johnson seemed unsure of the seriousness of the crisis even though other Europeans were getting attacked by a virus that started in China. Italy, for example, kept on warning the United Kingdom for over two weeks in advance. Our government didn't show any interest in these warnings. It was like we were their minions that were forced into a battle that we cannot arguably win at all. My manager and her husband decided to send me home on measurement of precaution.

As I was on the train travelling towards Seven Sisters to go back to Waltham Forest I wasn't feeling 100% well. It was like the universe was getting ready to cave in on me. Throughout my journey to my home it was like I was going to pass out.

As I was waking up from my sleep on Friday 20 March, that was when I was having symptoms related to Covid-19. My skin was cold like I was coming into habitation from a penguin igloo; my head was spinning like it was in a Beyblade battle getting attacked left and right. That was when I called my manager and told her that I was unable to go to work because I wasn't well; it was like the air in my proximity was poisoned.

So during the day I had to fight and claw through to survive the disease that was occurring. I had to cook and clean for myself to fight off this nasty virus in order to be alive. My mind started to think in overdrive about the people that I had cared for, which meant I had to enter into quarantine for fourteen days. It was like I was entering into the matrix where there is a beginning to an end. All I could do was to pray for hope.

For the moment, all I could do was to have a mask on anytime I decided to go out for either exercise or shopping, especially when I had a dusty, dry, irritable deep breath of a cough. So I decided to invest in some cough syrup and vitamin tablets in order to help solve my cough because it was also a part of the Covid-19 symptoms that the government has displayed, as well as the NHS guidelines, which became a reality when they decided to advertise on each station that was being broadcast on the television.

When I had my lunch, I went straight upstairs to shrivel up into a ball under my duvet sheets to keep my body warm at all costs. Beside my bed I had a bottle of water to prevent my cough from scratching my throat because it felt like I had cat fur in a ball wanting to come up me like a slimy slug. So as I was in my bed I was glimpsing into hope, pouring out my heart to the man above which is Jesus Christ, to protect me and my loved ones. But as it was the same result happening through to Saturday 21 March, my manager contacted me to see how I was coping under the circumstances. She was asking me how do I feel, am I eating properly, do I feel shortness of breath? All I replied back was that I had the cold and flu symptoms, and I'm doing very well and I'm taking natural remedies to help me fight this virus, and I'm eating very well, I was saying my breathing wasn't that bad, to the extent that the government had predicted it to be.

These symptoms were meant to cause our body into an overdrive like we were going to have a heartache or diabetes overdrive shock where your body isn't working to its full capacity.

The following day, which was Sunday 22 March, I had the same feeling but at a rate of feeling seven out of ten on the scale of not feeling well. Then this was the time when my mother decided to do a group WhatsApp call to me and both of my aunties to see how we were doing, because she had received news that the whole of the United Kingdom was entering into lockdown due to the level and numbers of Corona virus cases that were appearing across the entire National Health Service board. They were in total disbelief because the government didn't give them any warning at the time. So we as a family used the WhatsApp virtual group calling as a meeting format where we communicated each Sunday to do a spiritual reading, as well as a guideline of what to take and to see how we were coping on a daily basis. It was almost like guidance on how and what to do in order to get rid of any bacterial virus within our living environment.

So during the daytime when I started to move around the house I wasn't that bad. I still had a cough that was less tickly but more of a chesty dry cough that was becoming uncomfortable, especially when I was cleaning and doing my Sunday roast dinner. During dinner I would drink my ginger tea to help ease the irritation. Before I went to bed, I gargled my throat with warm salt water in order for me to have a good sleep.

When Monday 23 March arrived I woke up with a dry, chesty cough, so I decided to start my day with a drink of warm water and two slices of lemon to ease my throat as well as to boost my immune system. Then I had a bowl of Weetabix to help energize my day.

During that day I was drinking plenty of liquid as well as having a well-balanced health schedule, that consisted of exercise as well as fruits and vegetables. These nourishments were helping me throughout this pandemic because I felt that it was all about the survival of the fittest, especially when you consistently see the government statistic graphs. I felt like it was a wake-up call, due to the fact that it underlined the importance of us needing to take care of ourselves and that we need to care as well as cherish those around us who are vulnerable to being exposed.

Then on 24 March I spoke to my manager who told me to contact the NHS emergency number 111. At this point I never wanted to be part of their statistics, especially when the news or the advert was telling us what to do during the pandemic. At this moment in time I had to encourage myself to call the NHS number. The call itself was long-winded because it made me want to go and sleep. So whilst waiting for almost two hours someone eventually picked up the phone and spoke to me.

For that ten-minute conversation of questions and answers, I felt like an alien that already knew the answers to what they were going to recommend for me. The answer was cough mixture syrup for the treatment of a chesty cough, as well as to drink plenty of water.

But as the days were going by day to day I was rapidly making a good recovery. The dynamic of the surrounding was still the same especially when you went outside. My day felt like a hamster on a wheel, doing the same thing over and over again for a long period of time, and that is shopping for groceries as well as exercising. But some of my routines remained the same, like doing online stretches, and breathing techniques with my client twice per week because it was depending on his schedule as well. When we had finished what we did on our WhatsApp video call class, I would build conversations with him for between five to eight minutes in order to improve his confidence. These things that we were enlisting were to help calm down his anxieties.

As the months passed by and lockdown was easing, my manager and I put in a schedule for us to resume back to work for July and August. But everything had to seem reasonable in order to figure out what is this new normality, especially with these house bubble meeting guidelines for social distancing. But to see my manager as well as my client and family again felt wonderful because it was like we missed out on wonderful occasions. And then to catch up with our other VAC youth club members was also a good feeling, especially when we were exploring our adventures in different areas where we haven't been before.

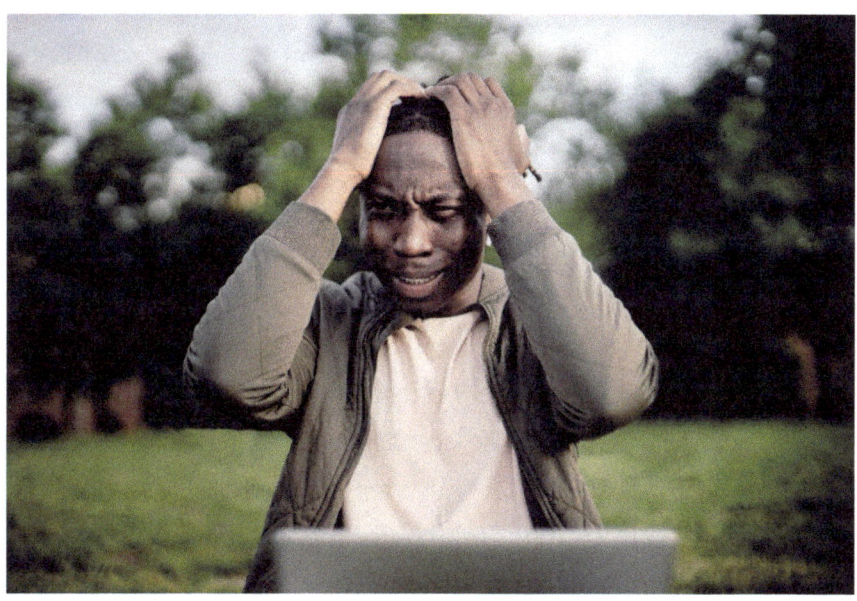

I'M AUTISTIC AND COVID HAS CLOSED MY FAVOURITE PLACES

Zeke's Covid Story told by his mother on his behalf

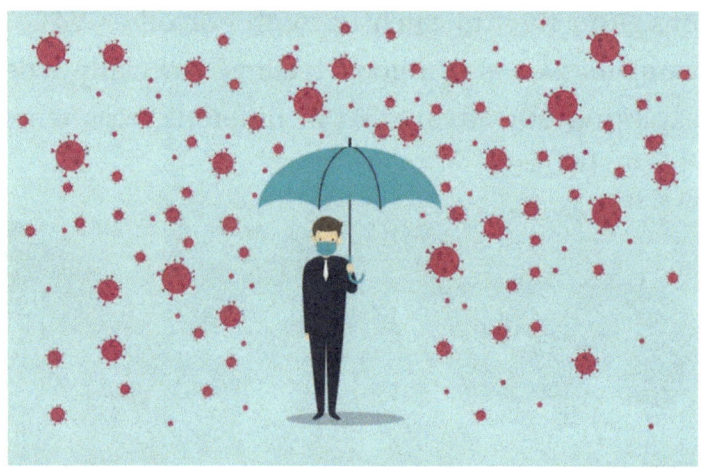

She finally came to the understanding that Covid-19 virus was much more serious than she believed it to be one week earlier, in early March 2020 when she first heard about it on the 6 o'clock news. New City College, Hackney was due to close for two weeks Easter holidays, from the week beginning 23 March and reopen the week beginning Monday 20 April 2020. However, my mother decided to withdraw me from college one week early from

Monday 16 March 2020. On Thursday 19 March she decided to dismiss Nathaniel, my support worker, from his duties with me until further notice as he was looking ill. She didn't stop there. That same day in the evening, when my father arrived home from work, she suggested to him that she did not think it was safe for him to be going into work as he uses public transport. After a short pause, to my surprise his response was, 'I don't think so either'. That was one of the easiest battles she'd won with my father. This response made her next step easier for her.

In her mind she began to think about what she needed to do to make this change in routine as straightforward as possible for me, knowing that I do not cope very well with changes. Weekly online FaceTime singing and piano lessons, weekly online Zoom physical exercise with Nathaniel, my support worker, weekly online Zoom Feldenkrais breathing and physical exercise with therapist Juliana, weekly online Zoom dance session with Haringey Shed, daily reading with me, daily walk around the block with my dad and me, daily jumping on the trampoline in the back garden and daily family time in the back garden, sunbathing and talking and eating, having time out on my phone, iPad and laptop, sleeping during the days if I felt the need to do so. As much as possible my parents encouraged me to watch programmes on the television with them. I was also given more choices than usual to bake and cook. My dad Zephie got me involved in digging the garden, mowing the lawn, planting plants in the garden and encouraged me to water them when necessary.

VELORA M. LEVY-SAILSMAN

I would frequently request reassurance about when certain shops and social provisions would reopen. Once I was given a time span when these would reopen I was happy with my parents explaining. I continued with my independent self-care such as taking a shower or bath twice daily and applying underarm deodorant after my first shower or bath of the day. I also helped freely to tidy my room and independently load my dirty clothes into the washing machine, adding detergent and clothes softener and choosing the correct washing programme. Under the guidance of my father, I did attempt to iron certain items of my clothing, which I enjoyed doing.

ZEKE'S FREQUENTLY USED COVID-19 WORDS

Covid-19   Corona virus   Pandemic   Social distancing

Wash your hands   Isolation   Wear a mask   Key-Workers

Doctors   Nurses   Hospital   Ambulance

Go for a walk   Take multivitamins   Eat your meals

Eat your fruits and vegetables   drink lots of water and juices

Shops are closed   Churches are closed   Youth club closed

Leisure centres closed   Swimming pool closed

Schools and colleges closed

Thank God for key workers

THE SPREAD OF COVID-19 AROUND THE WORLD

By Kenneth Osei-tutu

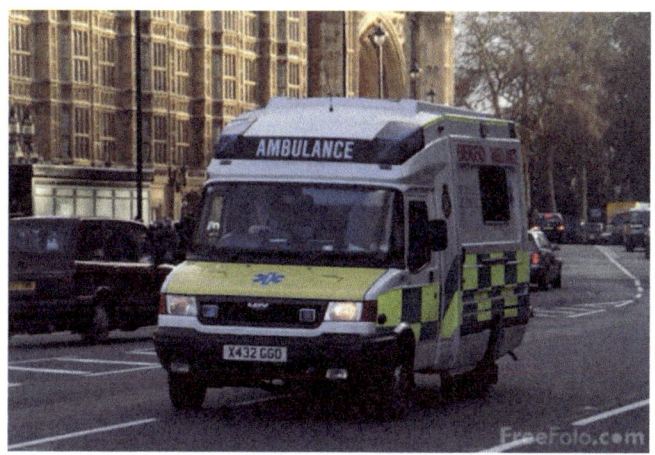

Some Covid-19 diagnosis patients recount their personal experiences with Corona virus and the care they received at Johns Hopkins Hospital in Maryland USA. They have recalled that one million people have now died from Covid-19 just over six months after the disease was declared a pandemic.

This is the story of how the virus spread around the world and some of the human tragedies behind the numbers. Boris

Johnson, the Prime Minister of the United Kingdom, said that come next Thursday 5 November there will be another lockdown of the country.

The virus can cause a range of symptoms, ranging from mild illness to pneumonia. The main symptoms of the disease are fever, a persistent dry cough, sore throat and headaches. In severe cases the victim will experience difficulties in breathing and death can occur.

Since social isolation was imposed I have received hundreds of telephone calls and messages, from friends and families with similar concerns. Everyone is terrified and stressed about future uncertainties. Some people including myself believe they have had symptoms of Covid-19 without any concrete confirmation because initially testing was not available to the general public. Some people ask about the risk of being patients with heart disease.

The human side of the pandemic is to discover the stories of the nurses, doctors and public health experts working on the frontline of the Corona virus pandemic.

The number of Covid-19 deaths has been shocking. Due to the number of deaths, starting back Monday 23 March and on Tuesday 24 March 2020 the British Prime Minster decided to impose the first national lockdown.

During these unprecedented times due to the Corona virus, young people find themselves stuck at their homes across the world. The unusual experience of self-isolation has significantly altered their lives and reality, bringing not only concerns and doubts but also opening doors for new opportunities and possibilities.

I ask myself the question, 'What future do I want after the Corona virus?' Young people will face the economic and social consequences for many years to come. They will no doubt have begun to develop their own thoughts about the future they want after the Corona virus fades away.

To engage in a constructive reflection UNESCO and TAKHTE are organising an essay contest for children and youths, entitled: Year one After Virus (AC). There will also be the 'Pan India Online Essay Contest 2020.'

MY COVID LIFE

By Herald Essuman

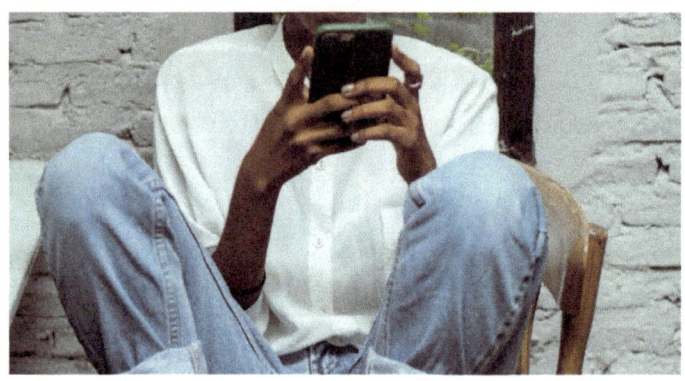

In March 2020 during the Covid-19 I had a bit of a cough. I had some Lem-sip to drink to help me get better. It was getting boring when I kept hearing about the virus on the news. I was getting fed up of hearing the same thing again so I turned the TV off. I spent my time going to Edmonton Green to do some shopping for the house.

I did some art using my phone and tablet to create something new. This was my first time hearing about Covid-19 in the UK. I didn't dwell on it because I didn't want to hear about it over and over again.

I spent some time in Stratford looking at some books in the book shop. I kept calm by not thinking about the virus. I went to the barbers to get my hair cut. I really enjoyed going out for some fresh air from my house. I also used my phone to do some word search to keep myself busy.

During the lockdown I went to the internet café to use the computer. The internet café kept me busy from the lockdown.

Mr Frank Odu was a family friend. He was 52 years old and out of work due to kidney problems and high blood pressure. He was already receiving treatment when suddenly he developed a cough, severe chest pains and shortness of breath. He was then admitted to hospital but died five weeks later.

The things I would normally do, like go to the cinema, Art box, the youth club and the library - I couldn't go to these places I like because of the Corona virus spreading around England and other parts of the world.

On 8 August I started going back to the Art box Centre and getting back to my art work I enjoy working on. After the lockdown was lifted I was able to go back to the barbers to get my hair cut. I was able to use the computer in the internet café and I was happy because the lockdown was lifted. During the summer as a team our youth club members planned a day trip to Trent Park and we had a picnic then we went for a walk around the park. We started attending the youth club again on Friday 4 September 2020.

I will feel disappointed if the virus continues spreading around winter time. I wouldn't be able to do the things I enjoy or like such as youth club, Art box, the barbers and going out to the cinema with friends. I will feel bored at home if there is another Covid-19 lockdown. I wish there wasn't Corona virus at all because it's spreading around the world and making people sick.

SAFE THROUGH THE STORM

By Valerie Ekoli on behalf of her son Kael

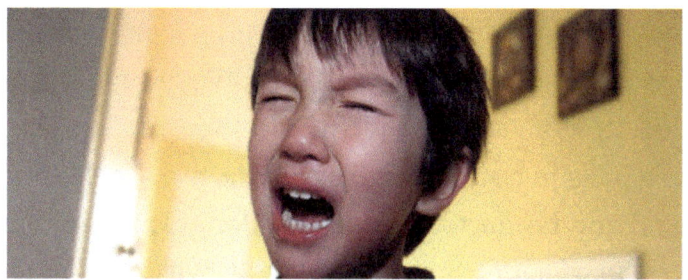

In March 2019 Kael started going through some traumatic time in his life. He became very unsettled in school, aggressive towards others and was finding it hard to cope with things around him. Life was dark and uncertain. But with God's help and the people involved in his care, like the professionals, he started making real progress again. He developed a new routine that he liked. He was getting dressed in the mornings, going to school in the bus, back etc. He was happy with that. Suddenly Corona virus came on the scene and everything changed. Lockdown happened and everyone was forced to stay home.

It was very difficult for my son. He did not cope well at all.

From day one he would cry a lot and have terrible meltdowns where he would throw himself onto the floor. He couldn't sleep well anymore.

We didn't know what to do to comfort him. He was pacing up and down in the flat. He was talking negatively to himself. It made him angry and always sends him into more meltdown. I had to be with him six days out of seven. The only day I could get a break from him was on Sundays when I was doing a long day at work. That was a frustrating time for my entire family, including his father and his two younger siblings. Before lockdown was eased we would take him to the park to kick some balls to burn off energy. It was fun. Kael would run in the field and he started sleeping better again at nights.

The only outside support we had was Kael's teacher, who was very supportive to me and my family. She would encourage me to look after myself. She would talk to Kael on the phone and on Zoom twice per week. This same social worker also called me twice per week to check on how things are going generally with the family. But there wasn't much she could do for us because of the lockdown.

The fresh breeze was very healing to Kael. During the hot summer we would open the patio door at home and the fresh breeze would come in. That was comforting for all the family. It kept Kael calm and helped him to cope well with the lockdown situation.

Eventually lockdown was over at last, thank God, after five months. Then suddenly Kael did not want to go out anymore so we spent the entire summer in the house. He father and I would take it in turns to take our other two children out. This was the only way we could get the other children to go outside, otherwise they would have to remain in the house all the time as well.

Now September arrived and it was time to return to school. Kael was transitioning to a new school and had not yet visited. It was a problem because he had not gone outside for five long months. Kael spent two and a half more weeks at home because he didn't want to go to school. His father and I simply could not get him out of the house. I had to keep cancelling the school bus service daily.

Eventually through prayer and the help of God we managed to get him out of the house. He's now in school and is settled despite having a new routine. He's doing well in school despite the challenges against him. He has ups and downs but things are looking better than before. Thank God that the second lockdown didn't last for very long. God be praised!

THE CORONA VIRUS AND MIRACULOUS ME

By Velora M. Levy-Sailsman

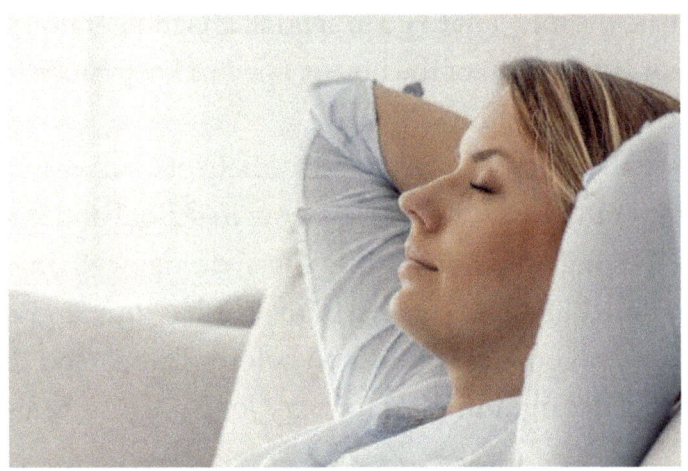

On 15 March 2020 the Prime Minister Mr Boris Johnson had announced the significance of a 3-week lockdown in order to stop the spreading of the Corona virus. This would mean that most businesses would be closed for this duration.

My dentist had by now cancelled my dental appointment for 20 March 2020 until further notice. I instantly had a thought about the seriousness of a tooth abscess which I'd developed since four weeks prior to the set date of my tooth implant appointment. I came to the conclusion that I could not endure the bad smell and pain in my mouth for any longer. So I make an immediate phone call to my dentist surgery in Finsbury Park, North London.

The receptionist was very considerate as she explained to me that my dentist has set aside Thursday the following week for emergency appointments and that he only had two appointment slots left, 8.45 am and 9 am. Giving consideration to my training and knowledge of the ins and outs of dental care I suggested to her I only needed a prescription for an antibiotic to drain the abscess from my tooth or gum. She proceeded to explain that the dentist will not write a prescription for any treatment without first examining the problem. I then suggested that I will have the 8.45 am appointment so she booked me into that slot.

Waiting a whole week to start the antibiotic treatment seems quite a long time so I was pleased when this day finally arrived. Equipped with my blue disposable face mask, my husband, my son Zeke and I travelled in our car for the 40-minutes drive to get to our dentist in Finsbury Park. We pulled up outside the surgery at exactly 8.40 am and I quickly made a call to the receptionist and announced that I'd reached the surgery.

At this time I was feeling quite light-headed, perhaps due to the gum infection and the infection from the abscess circulating into my blood stream. The receptionist came across a little abrupt and impatient with me, when I asked if the 9 am patient had arrived yet. She proceeded to explain that the 9 am patient would have to be seen before me as it would not be fair for her to be called after me as I was not yet there. When I explained to her that I was sitting in my car outside the surgery, and that I'd been doing so since five minutes ago, she was surprised and replied, 'So you're here? Well, you'd better come in and get seen to as the 9 am patient is not yet here.'

I went straightaway to the Reception, greeted the receptionist and announced my name to her. She replied and said, 'Your dentist is waiting for you so you can go in straightaway.' As I did the one-minute walk to my dentist's consulting room I instantly observed how clean and unusually quiet the space and seating area had been. My dentist's consultation room door was closed so I decided to take a seat on one of the chairs in the seating area.

Mr Mohammad did not allow me to be seated for more than thirty seconds when he opened his door and said, Mrs Sailsman, I'm ready for you so please come on in.' I felt an 'aura' of panic but I managed to thank him for seeing me despite the Covid-19 social distancing rule being already in place by the government. Both himself and his nurse were nicely and securely kitted out in protective equipment and were clearly ready to commence treating my abscess tooth problem. The dental nurse handed a protective blue apron to me which I took from her and quickly put on and proceeded to lay on the examination coach. My dentist then told his nurse to give me the protective glasses to wear also.

Instantly paranoia crept in my mindset when I gestured that she should put it away while explaining that, 'I don't know who was wearing it.' My dentist said, 'That's ok, you don't have to wear it.' He then proceeded to examine the abscess on my tooth. His comment was that 'it's a big one' and that 'it was covering two teeth'. He explained that he wanted to use his probe to pierce the gum as there was still some pus in the gum that needed to be drained out.

But I was adamant that he should leave things as it was because enough of the pus had already drained out into my mouth, which had a disgusting taste, and that I didn't wish for any more to leak out into my mouth as it would make me want to vomit again. I suggested that once I'd started to take the antibiotic that pus would naturally drain into my blood stream and then into my intestine for disposal as ammonia.

Surprisingly he agreed with me, then he said, 'It will.' He then proceeded to hand a prescription to me and said, 'Take care of yourself.' Then he added that he will send me a new appointment as soon as the social distancing rule and 'lockdown' measures got lifted. As I approached the reception desk to leave the surgery I cleansed my hands with some antibacterial gel which was put in place by the surgery staff. Then I went straight to the car where my husband and youngest son Zeke were still waiting in the car for me.

My husband asked if I'd got my prescription and I said, 'Yes'. The name of the medication I was given to treat my mouth abscess was Clindamycin. As soon as I returned home with it I spent time reading up about the possible side-effects. The most worrying side-effect for me was that it could cause breathing difficulties. Earlier I'd read up on another medication I was taking and noticed that this medication, known as Omeprazole, can also cause breathing difficulties. It was also registered in my brain that one of the classic symptoms of the Covid-19 virus is breathing difficulties. However, I proceeded to take both Clindamycin and Omeprazole but carefully made a written record of the time of day they were both taken.

After two days of taking the above two medications I noted that I was waking up in the early hours of the morning with rapid heartbeats and shortness of breath. On the third night of taking the medications the beating of my heart was disturbingly strong as I walked back up the stairs to my bedroom after using our downstairs toilet. I could hear my heart beating loudly and feeling it pressing against my chest and ribcage as if about to jump out of my chest.

It was now 5 am and I had to wait until 8 am when my GP's surgery would be open to seek further medical advice. I was too breathless to wait three hours so l anxiously discussed with my husband whether we should call our local 111 emergency service. After thirty minutes of deliberation my husband agreed to do so. This team of medical professionals did not attempt to pay us a visit until 3pm that same day.

My biggest worry was that I possibly had contracted the COVID-19 virus from my office, in which case, I would need to be hospitalised to receive the appropriate treatment. After completing their medical observation the two paramedics involved explained that based on my high oxygen level I did not have the Corona virus so they did not escort me off to a hospital.

The following day my breathing was getting worse so again, after much deliberation and prayers involving my husband, my husband again telephoned the 111 local medical emergencies. On this occasion two ambulances started pulling up outside our home within one hour, and on this occasion three paramedics appeared. Yet again they completed a thorough observation and again we were told that my oxygen level was too high and that it was not necessary for me to be admitted to hospital. We were advised to speak matters over with our GP because they are more likely to be of help to me.

At 4 pm we had a conference call with our locum GP who instructed us to discontinue Clindamycin medication, which she had by now replaced with Amoxicillin and it would be waiting at our pharmacy to be collected by my husband. Within an hour my husband had collected the prescription and I was now taking Amoxicillin and had also stopped taking Omeprazole. Omeprazole was a medication I had been taking for over two years to cure the reflux problems I have been experiencing for a number of years.

I wonder how many people have a testimony at the challenging corona virus time. I'd now started to take the Amoxicillin but my breathing difficulties appeared to be getting worse, particularly at night. I decided that I should sleep downstairs on the sofa so my husband's sleep would not be disturbed as he had become the person doing most of the chores around the home. He obviously needed to rest and maintain his health and strength.

I remember vividly using my laptop computer for a couple of hours before propping myself up on the cushions at one corner of the sofa to make myself comfortable enough to retire to try and have some sleep at about 11pm. I switched my laptop off and placed it on the shelf close by the chimney breast. Then I returned to the sofa and rested my back and my head against the cushions I had put in place earlier. I drifted off to sleep but woke up three hours later gasping for breath.

I looked over at my laptop and instantly noticed that the screen of the laptop was on and a picture of a lady could be viewed. With this shock l took a deep breath and managed to walk over to where the laptop was resting. I became curious to know about what was being shown on the screen of my laptop. I quickly noted that the triangular play button was showing. So I carried my laptop over to the sofa where I was resting earlier and decided to click on that play button.

To my surprise this was a short video from Boots the pharmacy. This video was describing two positions whereby the hands could be placed above the chest and resting on the forehead to assist with breathing difficulties. Immediately I tried out these exercises and noticed that the pressure I had previously felt in the middle of my chest and ribcage was greatly reduced. So I noted the time showing on the computer, it was now 3 am. I decided to replace my laptop on the shelf, have a sip of water, then used the toilet to empty my bladder and went upstairs to check if my son or my husband was still awake. In the back of my mind I was thinking that either of them must have returned downstairs to check on me to see if I was ok. When I observed the way both of them were fast asleep, I returned to the sofa to try and get some more sleep as I was feeling tired.

Firstly I placed my right hand on my forehead and it felt comfortable. Secondly I alternated with my left hand and it also felt comfortable. My lungs felt as if they were being lifted from my ribcage on which they had originally been attached and as a result preventing the oxygen from entering the lungs and also preventing the carbon dioxide from being released from the lungs. I was now able to inhale comfortably enough to have a sleep and did not awake until 8 am.

By this time both my husband and son were awake and up and having breakfast. I quietly walked to the bathroom to freshen myself up and changed into some daytime clothes. Whilst doing these activities my mind was pondering about how my laptop was switched on and I was certain that I had shut it down and turned it off before I went to sleep. When I returned to the dining area where my husband and son were sitting, finishing off their breakfast, I first of all asked them if they had slept well.

I stood beside them and asked if either of them had returned downstairs after going off to bed last night. My husband first replied, 'I didn't', then he said, 'Why do you ask?' I then turned to my son and said to Zeke, 'You came downstairs while I was sleeping and googled Boots the pharmacy, didn't you?' Zeke looked at me with defiance in his eyes and said, 'No!' Instantly I believed both of them.

I proceeded to explain to both of them how I woke up struggling to breathe then I noticed my laptop was on and it was displaying a video of a woman showing two positions we should place our hands if we're having difficulties breathing. Again my husband said it wasn't him and my son also replied that it wasn't him. I responded that this was a miracle from God and that he knew I was struggling to breathe and he came and helped me out.

Two days later another conference call with my actual GP and she has recommended Propranolol to reduce my heart beat by 40%.

This worked very well and my heart did not appear to be beating too fast and my breathing no longer seemed to be distressed. My GP explained that I was having a condition called 'panic attacks' which could have been brought on by me worrying too much. She wanted to know if I was worrying about anything in particular. I told her that I was worrying about catching the Corona virus and dying as a result of it. I also told her that I was worried about the fact that I may die due to the virus and leave my son behind with no one to give him the level of care that I have been giving to him.

The term 'Shielding of the vulnerable groups were introduced by the government. On 24 March Prime Minister

Boris Johnson declared a total 'lockdown' by the whole nation. We were instructed to remain at home with only members of our household. In my particular case this included me, my husband and our youngest offspring. We were given strict guidance in regards to how frequently we should go shopping and for a short walk around our local environment. All this we should do without speaking or coming into direct contact with other people.

The nation was given strict guidance by the Prime Minster when to do strict social isolation. If we had symptoms such as headache, a continuous cough and high temperature above 37.5 degrees centigrade then we should do social isolation within our homes to protect our resident family members from becoming easily exposed to the Corona virus. In this instance we should prepare a space in the family home where each family member would not come into direct contact with the family member who was showing signs of Covid-19. In our household that was easy to accomplish as there is a spare room which means each family member would be able to comfortably occupy a bedroom.

My biggest concern was the occurrence of a situation where both myself and my husband should contract the virus at the same time and our 21-year-old son, who has a diagnosis of autism, had to fend for himself. I had no further option than to suggest to my husband that we need the intervention of our God through Jesus Christ to help us through the situation in which we had found ourselves. We started to pray to our

God specifically to help us through this Corona virus time. God clearly answered our prayers because within a few hours my breathlessness had improved and twelve weeks on, in July 2020 we're all standing strong and feeling well in our mind and body. On reflection I'm almost certain that all three of us had experienced the Covid-19 virus. If that's the case, my husband and son have had it in a much milder form than me.

I've drawn this conclusion because during the second week of the lockdown in early April, all three of us experienced diarrhoea for over five days, but it did not affect our appetite. Our son also experienced vomiting, headaches and sweated at night for that same time duration. My symptoms included nausea and salivation of regular mucus, loss of appetite, feeling weak in my knees, breathing difficulties and breathlessness.

On two separate occasions we had no choice but to request help by dialling 111. On both occasions when the paramedics did their observations of me they had decided that my oxygen level was not low enough for them to have me admitted to hospital so they recommended that I should try and relax and breathe slowly and to contact my GP. This we did on at least 5 separate occasions, which was helpful to my medical and emotional situation.

Although the paramedics and my GP had reassured me that I did not have Covid-19, at the back of my mind I still think I had Covid-19 for 5 weeks, although the only supporting evidence was difficulties with my breathing, which at twelve weeks of lockdown was greatly improved and I was now sleeping much more comfortably at nights.

The term 'shielding' for vulnerable groups such as the elderly and clinically ill was also in place. These vulnerable groups were advised to remain at home for twelve weeks in order to isolate themselves from other people who may potentially pass the disease onto them. They were not expected to leave their homes at all and the only outside space they could use was their back garden or the balcony of their flats.

Although I was not really included amongst this 'at risk' group I decided to shield myself from the outside world for seven days before I started to join my husband and son on their daily short walks in our neighbourhood. Eventually when I decided I was well enough to go outside for this privileged walk with my husband and son. Each day before we left our home we would carefully put on our face masks and gloves as protection from the virus. This we did for eight weeks until the Prime Minister decided to lift some of his restrictions in early July.

Today we only wear our masks and gloves when we're entering an environment where it's impossible to maintain social distancing of two metres from the closest person to us. We have become very principled in our ways of keeping safe, such as washing our hands more frequently using anti-infection gel, changing our bedding weekly, cleaning work surfaces often, mopping all floors every other day using bleach and one other disinfectant and cleaning door handles weekly.

I now look forward most to seeing my two grandchildren and to having my hair attended to by my regular hairdresser. However, I have a burning desire to undergo the test for evidence whether I have the Covid-19 virus antibodies or not.

As a family we had in place coping strategies for the Covid-19 pandemic. Every Sunday at 2pm we had a Zoom chat with our two older children and their daughters. This was a delightful activity which involve catching up with events in our lives, laughter and seeing the progress in our two small granddaughters, Our eldest grandchild was now six years and five months old and now more willing and able to describe activities she has completed during the lockdown. Our second grandchild, on the other hand, was now three years old and was noticeably speaking much more clearly than before. It was surprising to hear that our two older offspring, had experienced breathing difficulties during the early stage of the lockdown.

At the end of the total lockdown we came to understand that my eldest son's fiancée, who is a midwife and is the mother of our first granddaughter, was tested for antibodies of the Corona virus in her body and the result was positive. At the end of the total lockdown we concluded that we've all had symptoms of the virus and have survived.

My weekly Egyptian dance session on Zoom with a professional dancer went well. Not only was I learning the routine of Egyptian dancing but I was getting exercise, and it was lovely speaking with a familiar person who had become a friend. I would tell her how I was feeling health-wise and she would give me tips on how to overcome certain physical health issues. Juliana later introduced Feldenkrais therapy exercises to me and I joined her group session for this. In addition it was lovely to see other people in the group and to have brief chats with them. Feldenkrais exercises have been helping me a lot with my breathing difficulties, anxieties and panic attacks.

To further help my breathing difficulties I also booked a weekly Facetime with a singing teacher. Paula has taught me how to fill my tummy with oxygen before singing and how to comfortably use this air for my singing. So I've learnt how and when to inhale and exhale while singing the whole song. She has taught me about singing from the belly and from the head and when to use the throat to do a vibrato. I particularly like the warm-up breathing exercises. They get the voice ready to start singing the song. Again, it was lovely to have Paula on board during the lockdown because she has taught me a specific exercise to strengthen the diaphragm and to expand the lungs and ribcage.

Also important to me was the daily phone call I would receive from my big brother who lives in Islington. I looked forward to him calling. Whenever I noticed a missed call from him I would phone him back straight away. Our conversations helped to build up my willpower for survival from the Corona virus pandemic.

As a family we agreed on Remedies we strongly believed would prevent the virus developing in our bodies.

VELORA M. LEVY-SAILSMAN

We had Our daily lemon drink Ginger, garlic and honey drink at nights for itchy throat. Gaviscon from the GP was used to clean out any 'muck or gunge' in the stomach and relieve heartburn
Daily vitamin D supplements
Multi-vitamins which included zinc and potassium
Eating more fruits and vegetables, Drinking more fruit juice and water Eating more healthy homemade meals Reading the bible and praying more regularly

Being Christians we strongly believe in Miracles from God. In mid-March 2021 during the second lockdown, I was invited by staff at Hadley Wood hospital to attend their hospital for an operation to remove some damaged arteries in my left leg. During preparation to go down to theatre the consultant explained to me that I have a clot also to be removed from the main vein in the same leg. This was truly a miracle to me because I was believing that the Corona virus was responsible for my breathing difficulties. But instead the origin of my breathing difficulties was due to the damaged arteries and clotted blocked vein I have been living with for forty years.

It was further explained to me by the Vascular surgeon that these factors were preventing oxygen from flowing freely around my body and to my various organs. Although these are life threatening conditions, I felt relieved that I did not have the corona virus after all. The most satisfying outcome was that this operation was performed under local anaesthetic using sedation, laser and suction. The operation to remove the clot which I was previously told could not be achieved has been successfully achieved. I regard this experience as a miracle from my God. I can now rest assured that I don't have to suffer the consequences of having had the corona virus.

VELORA M. LEVY-SAILSMAN

"The journey will be tiresome but the education phenomenal!"
Velora M. Levy-Sailsman
10.10.2021

The End